Cancer alternatives

What You May Know and What Your Doctor Will Not Tell You

DAVID ETHEREDGE

Table of Contents

THERAPIES AND PROTOCOLS...123

THE FOLLOWING BOOKS ARE RECOMMENDED..152

FOR FURTHER INFORMATION VISIT THESE WEB SITES.................................153

"Everyone should know that most cancer research is largely a fraud…" - Linus Pauling PhD (1901-1994) Two times Nobel Prize winner.

Why I Wrote this book?

One reason is because my wife of 21 years had long struggled with health issues, many of which were obvious signs of cancer. Note that there is a list of signs at the end of this book. She did not want to do either chemotherapy or radiation treatment and some of her cancer was inoperable. At that point in history, it was difficult to find information about some alternatives. I too, was plagued with a number of health issues but fortunately was blessed enough to not face terminal cancer 'yet', and hopefully never will. However, I am at serious risk because I worked as a chemist for a number of years. Chemists face a low average life span as well as a greatly increased risk of cancer. One reason why I quit and pursued a path in biomedical engineering.

I feel that if we had this information available to us in the early stages of her cancer, she could have survived much longer, so for that reason, I have put it here for you, the reader.

There is a high degree of skepticism and massive amounts of misleading information concerning alternative therapies for cancer. To that point, there are even people who are paid to misinform and mislead people away from alternatives. These people are usually referred to as trolls. One of their tactics is to find books on alternatives and give them bad reviews in an effort to dissuade people from reading.

Another effort is made through Cancer Organizations such as American Cancer Society which consistently refers to any alternative as unproven and potentially dangerous. However, you can see the truth in what they say by the number of studies on alternatives for cancer, practically none! In fact, the ACS keeps the bulk of the money that they receive for their own benefit, high salaries, self promotion, etc. Little of their money actually goes to research and almost all of that goes to profiting pharmaceutical companies. The ACS is not the only one in this respect. The Cancer fund raising industry is a massive scam in my opinion. Because I think that this is important, I will repeat and add to this later.

One cancer organization that does raise funds to study inexpensive alternatives is the AICR (American Institute for Cancer Research). What I recommend to anyone who wants to contribute to cancer research is to ask the question, how much does that cancer group provide to promoting "cheap, natural, alternative therapies" vs funding to "big pharma". Also, verify that those studies are not "hands on the scale" against natural and alternative.

I am not a medical doctor and am not an Oncologist so what I am providing is not medical advice but is only my thoughts based on my experience as well as some information gleamed from a number of sources. Also, there is little to no references in this book to sources. The information that I am providing is from multiple sources and most of what I have written is available over the Internet from at least 4 or 5 sources, so it is general information. There is a mention of a couple of studies and they were originally available on line but when I went back to check them the original pages were gone. At the next to the last section of the book, there are lists of recommended books and websites which may expand on what is written here.

This book is not intended to be a complete reference but is to help you learn the basics of what can be done and some information to help you along the way.

What a patient may expect

When facing cancer and possible death from cancer, patients expect their doctor to provide the best guidance and support. In this age of information, many have found that the information provided by the family doctor or the oncologist may be fairly limited or even seriously biased. Often, they will provide only information about traditional therapies while some others always want try the latest fad in chemotherapy or radiation. They appear to only know about chemotherapy, surgery, and radiation, having no interest in anything else. As a result, the oncologist will usually only offer chemotherapy, radiation, and surgery. Alternatives are rarely mentioned. Alternative therapies are even frowned upon and derided by organizations such as the American Cancer Society. Even after being proven wrong, the ACS does not apologize or even acknowledge its erroneous postings and publications. As their normal mode of operation is to state something along the lines of 'this substance has not been proven to reduce or cure cancer', while they fail to mention that they have never provided any funding whatsoever to try to find out if any alternative would be even the slightest bit helpful in fighting cancer. Almost all funds raised by the ACS is spent on trying to raise more money and the very high salaries to the upper management and only after that is any spent on drug, radiation, and surgical research. At the very best it might go so far as to say that in some limited cases the alternative might have some limited benefit. The whole point is that the American Cancer Society and others are fund raisers for the pharmaceutical companies and is a propaganda machine against any therapy that would compete or reduce the profit coming from their creations. There are other, more progressive organizations that raise funds for alternative therapies as well as for pharmaceutical agents. One of these is the AICR, the American Institute for Cancer Research. The AICR invests into research for alternative and nutritional therapy in addition to traditional therapies. Before you invest your money in any charitable organization, investigate into where their funds go and how much actually gets spent on research. You can even earmark your funds to investigation of a particular therapy.

It should be noted that most oncologists would not accept chemotherapy for treatment if they were found to have cancer. Many would also not accept most of the radiation therapies. The cancer patient should also consider the profit motive. The fact is that chemotherapy often generates $10,000 per treatment or even more. The oncologist makes a lot of money from providing chemotherapy, radiation, etc. Many of the chemotherapies and radiation treatments that they offer cause new cancers later in life and other health problems as well. Chemotherapy and radiation can both destroy many of the bodies organs, damaging the heart, liver, kidneys, and even damaging the brain and nervous system. They almost always damage the bone marrow, which produces your new blood cells. In fact, one unreported statistic is that chemotherapy often kills, even as a result of only one treatment. This statistic is well hidden. In one survey, it was found that only about one-third of physicians and oncology nurses would have consented to chemotherapy for non-small-cell lung cancer. In another survey, it was found that of 118 Canadian doctors who treat lung cancer, only 16% would want chemotherapy for symptomatic metastatic bone disease. Another study found that about 1 in every 4 of such deaths had either been sped up or even caused by chemotherapy. The studies findings also included the discovery that 2 out of every 5 of the patients had suffered significant poisoning from their treatment. This actually is not surprising because in order to have any effect on cancer, chemotherapy must be extremely toxic. It is like drinking or being injected with the most horrendous poisons, hoping that it kills the cancer before it kills the patient. Only the strongest and healthiest will survive and even then, their future health will be seriously impaired as a result. In another review of 600 cancer patients in Britain who died within 30 days of treatment has found that one in four of the deaths was either caused or hastened by the chemotherapy. The results of chemotherapy are often liver damage, kidney damage, damaged immunity, and cellular aging. Another problem is that chemotherapy does cause brain damage and loss of memory. Those who survive the chemotherapy may be grateful to still be alive but may have to deal with years of pain, anguish, or even more deadly recurrences of cancer.

Before we go further, I would like to introduce a few important points about cancer and cancer treatment.

Some truths about cancer

In the 1950s when I was growing up, cancer was rare and you had about a 1 in 30 chance of developing cancer in your lifetime. Now the risk is about 1 in 2, in other words, half of all the people living in the U.S. are expected to develop cancer during their lives. This should bring into immediate question, WHY?

Lie number 1! Because we are living longer ????

In 1950 men lived on the average 65.6 years and women lived 71.1 years, in 2016 it was 76.3 for men and 81.2 for women, if the statement was true then the cancer rate for men younger than 65 years would remain at 1 in 30 and the cancer rate for women younger than 71 years would remain the same 1 in 30 as it was back in 1950. We all know that this is obviously wrong and a complete lie, on top of that, if it was true that cancer has increased because we live longer, then why has the cancer rate skyrocketed in children, including young children? Really, is it because children are living longer?

Lie number 2! We have reduced and eliminated so many other causes of illness ????

Seriously? While sanitation and good habits have helped reduce certain diseases and forms of illness, that would serve only to reduce those causes but not to increase the incidence of others, unless ... unless some of the methods of disease reduction such as vaccinations and medications are actually causing cancer.

Well, yes, it is a major problem that many medications and vaccinations as well are not tested long term to verify that they do not cause cancer. A carcinogen can take many years to cause cancer growth. There are many new antibiotics that are known to cause a wide range of adverse reactions in the short term but there are NO long term studies to determine whether or not these might cause cancer, auto-immune disorders or possibly other conditions such as MS, ALS, etc., also, other things may be causing cancer such as steroids that are given to reduce pain, swelling, and inflammation. Even greater is the concern over vaccinations, which is some cases have actually been proven to cause cancer in humans. In fact, the vaccine producers are so aware of this problem that in the US and in many other countries as well, they have asked for and received immunity from legal recourses.

So, if it is not a problem of living longer and not a problem of reduced deaths from other causes, WHY?

Lie number 3, When doctors start treating you for cancer and you ask 'Why did I get cancer?' Their common reply is 'we do not really know'.

That is nothing but an escape or cover up. The causes of cancer have been known since the 1930's when Otto Warburg discovered that cancer cells fueled their growth by consuming enormous amounts of glucose (blood sugar) and breaking it down without oxygen. It was also later discovered that in humans, insulin levels were also a major participant in the process of cancer growth, whereas, normal cellular growth used a different process where oxygen was used to oxidize smaller amounts of glucose to energy in a much more efficient process. While this is somewhat simplified here, it is the basis for the difference between normal cellular metabolism and that of cancer growth.

Lie number 4, When asked 'should I change my diet?', most oncologists reply just eat a normal diet!

The problem here is that through their ignorance about the relationship between nutrition and the development of cancer, they do not even know that the actual foods that you are eating may be part of the cause of the development of cancer. As noted above, cancer thrives on sugars and any food that you eat which may increase the levels of blood sugar can also increase cancer growth and cancer survival while at the same time, reducing your chance of survival as well as reduce your general health. There are foods that should be avoided which are classified as high glycemic index foods and can even include white bread, potatoes, and many other forms of starch or sugar.

Cancer may start in the body of any person, but if a person is perfectly healthy their cancer is quickly found and destroyed by the immune system. This is important!

True! I repeat, if a person is perfectly healthy their cancer is quickly found and destroyed by the immune system!

Herein lies much of the difference, and doctors are almost completely uneducated in this respect. A healthy immune system will quickly dispatch any developing cancer. The great percentage of doctors do not even realize that an increased blood sugar depresses the immune system! Also, the immune system is depressed by many other things such as improper flora in the intestines, improper levels of minerals such as selenium, magnesium, boron, or even iodine in the body. Even proper levels of Calcium and magnesium are critical to good health, whereas such things as mercury from dental amalgam or vaccines can seriously suppress the immune system, as can aluminum from vaccines. Even fluoride from drinking water or toothpaste can have a very negative effect on the immune system as well as some of the above are also related to mental health issues.

There are only a very few cancers that chemotherapy actually is helpful with and some studies show that chemotherapy has a mortality rate as high as 50 percent from the chemotherapy alone. One case that I know of personally was diagnosed with cancer and was given 12 to 15 months to live if she did nothing. She was convinced to take chemotherapy, did 1 round and died in just over 3 months. The chemotherapy definitely killed her but statistically she was listed as a cancer death in the group that did not do chemotherapy. This is one of the slights of hand that they use 'fingers on the scales' to make chemotherapy appear better than it actually is. To be placed into the chemotherapy group, they must be able to finish the chemotherapy. In this way, only the strongest go into the chemotherapy group. And even though someone started chemotherapy but could not finish it, they are placed into the 'other' group, 'did not do chemotherapy' to make the non-chemotherapy group look worse and appear to have a higher mortality. Also, if they determine that a person is too weak or too sickly to do the chemotherapy, or if they are not likely to be successful, they are told that chemotherapy is not an option for them and they get placed in the non-chemotherapy group. If you do not see the pattern of fingers on the scales, then read again.

Much of the same is true for radiation therapy.

Lie number 7, 'Once the therapy is over, you will recover and there is a reduced chance of recurrence.'

If you take chemotherapy or radiation, odds are that you will never completely recover from it, if nothing else, both chemotherapy and radiation will at least compromise if not destroy your immune system. This not only opens the door for cancer to return, but numerous other health issues as well. If you take chemotherapy and the cancer goes away for 5 years but you die of cardiac failure or pneumonia or even the flu, it shows as a cure but it does not show as a chemotherapy caused death. The same is true if you later suffer from either liver failure or kidney failure, no blame on either the chemotherapy or on the radiation.

So, does chemotherapy ever work? Actually, there are a few cancers that chemotherapy can work for but you still face the same risks of death and injury or even long term problems such as organ failure. Also, it should be noted that there are also some people that fare much better. These are the people that go the extra distance and DO NOT follow the doctors orders to eat normally. These are the people who swap to eating the proper vegetables and fruits, who do 1 day or 2 day water fasts, who juice only low glycemic vegetables, especially things such as broccoli, kale, wheat grass, sprouted alfalfa, small amounts of carrot peels (remember that carrots have more sugar than many other vegetables and the same with beets). Do not completely ignore meats, eggs, and fish. All have nutrition that is valuable to the body that can NOT be obtained from any vegetable source.

Have all of your vitamin levels and trace minerals checked. Have your hormone levels checked. Why? Hormones in the proper levels do boost immunity. If you are over 40, especially look at your Melatonin levels and your DHEA-S levels. In fact, if you are younger that that and are struggling, check them any how.

The Most important thing that your doctor probably does not understand?

Doctors, with the very little knowledge that they are given on nutrition, diet, and health (that is right, doctors are not actually taught what good health is.) are only told that these things have a normal range. They are NEVER taught about OPTIMUM health, OPTIMUM nutrition, OPTIMUM hormone levels. Really, isn't that what you really want and need? Optimum health for optimum lifespan!

So, what works against cancer?

If you take a look at societies and cultures around the world, there are some specific groups that have lower cancer rates than others. What do these people do to reduce cancer occurrences? One notable habit is monthly water fasting for a full 24 hours. Another is 12 hours minimum between the last food at night and the first food in the morning (NO midnight snacks), Fresh home grown foods, spicy diet with lots of peppers, onions, tumeric, etc., non-processed foods, and water that comes from a good clean source with a good mineral content.

As a note, one of the things that people often discuss about chemotherapy is that it tends to make them too sick to eat for a day or two. Perhaps this is one of the reasons that it works for the ones who do have success, forced fasting?

So, where do the statistics come from that the doctors use to justify the use of chemotherapy to "cure" cancer? First, is chemotherapies definition of cure, living at least 5 years and 1 day after diagnosis and not having a discernible tumor. According to this definition, the cure rate can continuously improve without ever having an actual improvement in health just by discovering cancer earlier. This is literally the basis of increased cancer survival today. On top of this, certain individuals and groups with lower than normal survival expectancy can be eliminated from the statistics. Another trick is to include things such as easily curable forms and even precancerous conditions that might lead to cancer in only a percentage of cases. One of the most absurd manipulations is the exclusion of patients that become too sick to complete chemotherapy or even patients who die during treatment. In order to be considered as part of the statistics, the patient must survive the chemotherapy or not be counted at all. On the other hand, the comparison group (those who do not get chemotherapy) includes those who are too sick or weak to start chemotherapy. A person who has cancer so bad that there is little or no chance of survival is placed in the group that does not receive the chemotherapy in any study. These are the people who get left in the control group but eliminated from the test group. According to a study by a group in Australia, The overall contribution of curative and adjuvant cytotoxic chemotherapy to 5-year survival in adults was estimated to be only 2.1% in the USA. This fails to recognize that at 6 years, the numbers flip and there are more people alive that refused chemotherapy than those who accepted it. This is the number that oncologist do not want to talk about. It shows without a doubt that chemotherapy takes lives and shortens life expectancy. There is an additional factor that may be used to skew the numbers. The actual data used for the chemotherapy group is only those who are able to complete the chemotherapy. If a patient gets too sick to complete the chemotherapy, then they are removed from the chemotherapy group and placed into the group which did not complete chemotherapy which they try to make you think is the group which did not take any chemotherapy. It is actually composed of patients that were too sick to take chemotherapy as well as those who failed to complete the chemotherapy due to one reason or another. Either way, the data that they provide is misleading and is intended to convince you to take some seriously damaging but highly profitable poison. Just another way of putting the fingers on the scales.

Why do you have Cancer?

Ask your doctor why you have cancer, what causes it. Many do not know or will not say and how can you trust someone to cure something that they do not even understand the cause. It is even more important that you understand that cancer is not a disease, it is a symptom of a greater overlying condition. This is why cancer often returns even after chemotherapy, etc. have supposedly beaten it. Those who go beyond the standard therapies and include nutritional and alternative therapies live longer and have a higher success rate. I would also suggest that those who avoid chemotherapy, radiation, and radical surgery and use only nutritional and alternative therapies often have the longest life expectancy and success rates. Medical professionals will quickly question these statements claiming that there are not any scientific studies to support them. Medical science does not study alternative therapies and they are often not reported. People who do alternatives generally do not tell their doctors. Doctors in general do not ask. Some doctors even refuse to see patients that do alternatives. Doctors are also poorly educated in nutritional science and many have almost no education in this field. If you ask them what you should eat, they say "eat normal" or eat a regular diet. This is like they are saying, "eat the same things that caused your cancer in the first place".

They are completely ignorant of the fact that there are some foods that actually fight cancer better than the poisons that they propose to give you., and other foods actually feed and grow cancer. When you ask these doctors, they will often respond that they do not know anything about nutrition, supplements, or alternatives.

Alternatives to standard cancer treatment

What are the alternatives to the standard suggested treatments? The first necessary action is to learn what the medical profession knows or understands. Have the doctor discuss your blood tests, urine test, and scans with you. Learn every detail about your condition. Nobody, not even your doctor, will have the devotion or will produce the effort to find the important details that will shed light on why you have cancer and how you can eliminate it. You, in the long run, are your number on advocate and in order to best help yourself, you need to know and understand what you are dealing with. There are test results that tell a lot about your general health and probable survival that may be more important than cancer size, type, and location. There are some tests that doctors do not even think of ordering. Doctors rarely order tests such as blood pH, serum magnesium, free vitamin D in your plasma, or hormone levels, but they can be valuable clues to the cause and outcome of your cancer. When you read your blood test results, if there is something that you do not understand, keep asking questions until you do have an accurate understanding. Following that, it is important to learn about the many things that the medical profession cannot or will not do or things that they do not bother with that might make a difference. Medical doctors are constrained by certain rules and requirements and some treatments are limited as to who may be eligible to receive them. Your doctor is also probably under the extensive influence of pharmaceutical companies, which actually provide a significant portion of the doctor's income. As a result, the doctor may choose therapies that benefit the pharmaceutical companies, the clinic, and the doctor more than they benefit the patient. Also, there are some therapies that must be requested because your doctor can not offer them. An example is Laetrile, vitamin B17, which must be requested by the patient. The doctor will probably respond that Laetrile is not legal in the US, but it is legal by court order. No matter what they tell you, in the U.S., it is your God given right to use the herbs of the earth and you can not be legally denied. Finally, it is important to look at long term cancer survivors to see what they have done to continue living where others have failed. This includes looking at things they may have done beyond normal therapy, including lifestyle changes. One thing to remember especially if your condition is considered terminal is that it is your health and you have a right to make your own decisions. This includes rejecting treatments that you do not want and requesting treatments that may not be approved. If your doctor does not want to cooperate, find another or get an attorney to help. Your doctor may tell you that these alternative therapies are not proven. You may respond in like that they have not been disproved either, despite many attempts to do so. Mainstream cancer therapy considers alternatives to be such a threat that those who profit from chemotherapy will go to great lengths to invalidate alternative and nutritional therapies. In reality, many cancer survivors credit the alternative therapies that they secretly followed for helping stop their cancer.

What Is Cancer

While cancers vary in origin, symptoms, and mortality, what is known about cancer is that it is a loss of genetic control of certain cells within the body. As the body normally develops, various genes inside of each cell are selectively turned on or off according to the bodies needs. Some of these genes contain codes designed to cause cell growth and cell replication and these genes are normally regulated in such a way as to provide a controlled growth and replacement of aging cells. Cancer cells frequently appear in the body but they are normally found and removed by the body's defenses. Sometimes, if the cancer has grown to big for the body to defeat, the body will encapsulate the cancer to keep it from spreading. This is how a cancer turns into a tumor. Once the integrity of the tumor is violated, as may happen during biopsy, or by being mashed when doing a breast exam or during a mammogram, the cancer is able to spread or metastasize throughout the body. It is the defined function of the body's immune system to kill and remove aberrant cells and materials such as cancer from the body. This includes tracking down and killing cancer cells. Cancer only thrives when the immune system is impaired. You should be aware of this important fact when considering any medical treatment. Chemotherapy almost always damages the immune system and many of the chemicals used in chemotherapy are mutagenic, that is that they produce new cancers. Radiation causes new cancers as well as damaging the immune system. Surgery is also a risky endeavor, especially in this age with antibiotic resistant bacteria and other illness causing agents that are common in hospitals. Of the three, surgery, chemotherapy, and radiation, surgery is the one option that is the most successful in saving lives, provided that surgery is done at the same time as the biopsy, reducing the risk of metastasis. Sadly, surgery only eliminates the obvious tumor but can not remove any cancer cells that may have spread. Also, surgery does not remove the conditions that caused the cancer to begin with.

While it has been scientifically shown since the 1930's, what many scientists and doctors do not fully recognize is why and how these cancerous cells fail to remain in control of their own natural processes and why the immune system fails to recognize and destroy them. According to current doctrine, these cells for some unknown reason just loose the ability to regulate themselves and the only way to stop this unregulated growth is to kill the renegade cells with harsh poisons and dangerous radiation. Both of these treatments cause serious damage to the immune system as well as the other body organs and either of these treatments can cause death. Radiation does effectively kill cancer cells as well as normal cells but in the long run, it is almost guaranteed to create new cancers. In fact, radiation, from x-rays to radio-active fallout to even some radio waves, actually directly causes some cancers. Doctors cover this up by saying that the cancer came back rather than admitting that they caused new cancer. Radiation also weakens the immune system and causes extensive damage to other cells in the body. Most chemotherapy is nothing but taking poisons in hope that they kill cancer cells more than they will kill normal healthy cells. Sadly, most chemotherapy causes new cancer growth in many cases and destroys normally healthy cells in the body in other cases. Again, chemotherapy almost always damages the immune system and other organs as well. Perhaps it is time for health professionals to rethink their approach to cancer causes and treatments.

Cause of Cancer

Toxic Chemicals

It is well known that exposure to certain chemicals can cause cancer to increase in occurrence. Many household cleaners, polishes, etc contain substances that are known to cause cancer. Even stronger cleaners and disinfectants are used on the farms where our food is grown, in the processing plants where it is packed, in the trucks where it is transported, and even many boxes that are used to pack the food. Pesticides and herbicides such as Roundup are known to cause cancer and they are sprayed on many crops. Even the FDA which is supposed to protect us supports many of these contamination sources in order to reduce bacteria, fungi, and other pathogenic organisms.

Radiation

Exposure to radiation can increase cancer occurrences. The incidence of cancer in the throat, mouth, and neck is directly related to the number of dental X-rays that a person has had. A single CAT scan can actually provide radiation equal to a thousand single X-rays. A PET scan is actually putting radioactive chemicals into your body. The nuclear testing of the 1950's and 1960's have exposed all of us to some increased radioactive isotopes that are known to increase cancer risk. These dangerous forms of common elements are in our food, water, and in the dust in the air and it will be for sometime to come.

Foreign organisms

The presence of certain parasites in the body can increase the occurrence of some cancers. There are several viruses such as HPV and some bacteria that are known to increase cancer risk. None of these, however, can be shown to always cause cancer. Sometimes, there is not any obvious reason for cancer to occur. This does not mean that there is not a cause, only that the cause is not obvious.

Why does cancer occur in some individuals but not in others? Is there a nutritional reason or is it genetic? Is there a problem with the immune system? Could it just be chance, bad luck? People around the world can get cancer, however, it is far more prevalent in the U.S. and some other industrial nations. Some would have you believe that this is because we live longer, forget it, the U.S. is 43rd in the world in life span. There are some things that we can look at to help us understand why cancer is so prevalent in the U.S. as compared to some other countries. Perhaps it may be because we are the most vaccinated country in the world? Is it because we use so much plastic where other countries do not? Is it partially due to excessive chlorine and fluorine in our water? Is it because we inhale more gasoline fumes than people in other countries?'Is it because we get too little vitamin D because we are inside almost all day? Are we missing some other important nutritional substance such as vitamin B17? Is it because we consume too much meats that have been raised with chemicals, artificial hormones, and unnatural nutrition? Is it because we consume too few vegetables and fruits or because the vegetables and fruits are low quality? Is it because we get insufficient exercise? All of the above are sure to contribute to our cancer epidemic along with many other factors. The truth is that cells fail and become cancerous almost daily and it is a failure of the immune system to catch and eliminate these aberrant cells. The immune system is one link to preventing cancer and fighting it that we have much control over. In reality, cancer is the result of the weakest link or the result of the weakest links.

The immune system failure

The one thing that is well known is that it is the job of the immune system to protect the body from the spread of cancer and normally it does so very well. It has been stated that the average American develops cancer at least 10 times over their lifetime but never knows it because the immune system takes care of it. It is only when the immune system fails to effectively do its job that cancer grows and spreads. It is a sad note that most of the therapies offered by medical practice today actually suppress or even destroy the immune system or at least important parts of it. The first question to ask about any therapy is "how will it affect my immune system?" If the answer is in any way negative then the best advice is, that therapy should not be accepted unless the situation is dire and the threat is imminent. Preserve and boost your immune system, as it is the one best chance for beating cancer and long term survival. New cancer cells are produced in the body nearly every day from the day that we are born and most likely from early gestation. The immune system is designed to recognize and destroy these aberrant cells. It is only when the immune system fails that cancer grows and spreads. If the immune system is not working properly, nutrition may be one of several factors that need attention. It is definitely known that the number one change associated with cancer remission is a change to a diet of fresh raw natural fruits and vegetables. However, as you will read later, it matters most of all the difference is in which fruits and vegetables, when, and how much.

Cancer and physiology

In choosing a path to fighting cancer, a good place to start is by examining the physiological changes associated with cancer.

Acid-Alkaline pH balance and Cancer

The question of alkalinity in the body is an important one but, it is not ALL about acid, so I would like to add some clarification here.

When is acid acid?

In biochemistry, an organic acid is a compound has a COOH radical attached. This makes it work as an acid but not necessarily strong. An example is alpha lipoic acid (ALA) and another is acetic acid (vinegar). Because of the weakness of organic acids, it would take massive doses of fatty acids to make even a small effect on pH. It does not take much baking soda to neutralize a lot of vinegar and baking soda (sodium bicarbonate) is actually a very weak alkali..

So, what is an alkali?

The opposite to an organic acid is an amine which has either a NH2 radical attached or a RNH radical. Ammonia is NH3, a strong alkali but amines are not as strong. As a note, amino acids have both -COOH and -NH2 terminations.

What is this acid-alkaline balance about?

Acid-alkaline balance is critically important in the physiologic function of the body and being either too alkaline or too acid can quickly kill you. As a point, if the blood gets too acidic, it causes kidney failure and other organ failures as well. This can be caused by issues such as excessive Lactic acid in the blood from too much strenuous exercise. Lactic acid is produced in the body at anytime that the cells do not get enough oxygen for their needs. This can take place in respiratory failure, extreme exercise, or in cancerous growths.

pH regulation

The body works hard to keep the pH at the right level and will sacrifice bone or anything else to regulate the pH between 7.25 and 7.45. when it can not do this, organ failure will quickly follow. If an acid condition occurs and is found in time, IV-bicarbonate is given to buffer the blood pH. Doctors and medical professionals will say that 7.25 to 7.45 is the range that the body regulates the blood pH to and that outside of this range you will die. Yeah, sure, but why do they not get that if the blood pH drops to 7.27 that you are near death? The regulation of pH is not doing what is needed for some reason. Why do they not get that optimum is 7.38 and that is where almost every function in the body works best? Being too acid, even below 7.30 impairs proper immune function, respiration, and many other physiological functions as well.

Doctors and health

Those doctors studied the same biochemistry that I did but they do not see the forest for the trees being in the way. For a long time I have pounded out the idea that for health and longevity, **you need everything to**

be optimum for your body. Optimum blood pH, optimum hormones, optimum nutrition, optimum environment, optimum exercise results in optimum immunity.

Saliva pH

So, what does all of this have to do with saliva pH? Saliva pH needs to be alkaline because that the optimum pH for the main enzyme, amylase, is 6.8 to 7.0. You might say wait a minute, that is slightly acid, and you are right but the sugars released from starches by the amylase tends to lower the pH. So saliva should start out with a pH of about 7.4. So, what does it mean if the saliva pH is below this, especially if it is acid? It basically may mean that the salivary gland may not be pulling enough alkalinity from the blood or that the blood is actually pulling alkalinity from the salivary glands as well as from the rest of the body. If the saliva is acid, it definitely is an indicator that there is something wrong.

Urine pH

As for urine pH, the kidneys are a major regulator of the blood's biochemistry, not just pH. The kidneys are a pump that is designed to regulate the elimination of unwanted materials from the blood and as a result from the body. A major part of this is the removal of acidity from the body, if for no other reason, self protection. Acidity can quickly destroy the kidneys. So, guess what? If your urine is seriously acidic, then your kidneys are being bombarded with acid and are not working in optimum conditions. If the urine pH is only slightly acidic then that may not be an issue but below about 6.6, I would be seriously concerned.

Checking the pH

It is best to check urine and salivary pH first thing in the morning, just after waking, before drinking or eating, do not even take any medication. Also, if you wake in the middle of the night, it is best not to eat or drink then either. The reason? both food and water consumption in any form affects the urine pH for up to several hours after. Even if you take medicines there will be some affect. There are many disagreeing sources as to optimum urine pH but I believe that 7.3 to 7.4 is optimum but I would not panic if it was 6.8 at times. If the early morning urine pH dropped below 6.5 for any length of time, again, I would become very concerned. There are pH kits available from many sources at reasonable prices.

Case notes

As I already mentioned, I lost my wife back in 2006 as a result of cancer pain medication. At the time she was diagnosed in the final late stages of cancer, her urine pH had dropped to about 5.4 to 5.6. We fixed her diet and nutrition, her pH came up but not to normal. She started recovering and outlived her doctor's last projection by between 4 to 8 times - no chemo but she did later take some alternative treatment from the Burzynski Clinic. Her oncologist had very stodgily given her 2 to 4 weeks to live in early March 2006. She did suddenly pass and it was realized that her doctor changed her pain medication to something that was marked on the front of her folder Do not prescribe, allergic (in big red letters). The point of the fact that she was making recovery is that the urine pH makes a big difference.

Cancer deaths and pH

Most cancer patients actually die from organ failure. Kidney failure and liver failure often occur first. I would strongly suggest that because of all that these people have been through, their ability to regulate the blood pH fails, and the organ failure follows shortly. For this reason, keeping the pH at a good level is critically important.

pH rules

Dr. Simoncini of Italy discovered that he could stop many cancers with simple baking soda treatments. The very point of this, that even if not 100 percent effective, it is a treatment that only costs a few dollars when compared to Oncology treatments that cost hundreds of thousands. There goes the medical professions profits!

Alkaline water concentrate

by David Etheredge

I use the following in 1 gallon of spring water to make a concentrate:

1 tbsp pickling lime (calcium hydroxide)

1/2 tbsp Epsom Salt (magnesium sulfate)

1/4 tsp no-salt (potassium chloride)

1/4 tsp baking soda (sodium bicarbonate) I originally used Sea Salt for the sodium but baking soda provides

additional alkalinity..

vigorously shake to dissolve each time that some is used as follows:

Do not take this straight or undiluted!

I take 1 tbsp of the concentrate and dilute to 1 gallon of water.

I drink 2-4 glasses of this every day depending on my needs. Do not drink too much. Also, take vitamin D3 along with K2-MK7 to help with calcium absorption and utilization. Reduce this amount if you experience any abnormal health signs and stop when you pH readings are outside of the acid range.

My early morning urine pH was very acid (approx. 5.8) a year and a half ago (2006) and the alkalizing diet was not working fast enough.

My pH was quickly within normal range using this alkaline water. It is important to use care not to over-alkalize as this can be as bad as being too acidic. Get close to normal then reduce consumption of alkaline water.

Another important element is iodine which is best painted on the bottom of the feet (Lugol's Iodine). Also look into sulfur compounds and selenium sources such as MSM.

More discussion of pH

One physiological condition that occurs with cancer is a noticeable drop in body pH balance. The pH or hydrogen potential is a measurement of acidity or alkalinity and ranges on a scale of 0 to 14 with 0 being the most acid and 14 being most alkaline. A pH of 7.0 is considered to be neutral, neither acid nor alkaline. Stomach acid is normally pH 1.0 or lower in order to properly digest proteins. The body pH is monitored as blood pH, urine pH, and saliva pH. The body must regulate the pH of the blood very tightly or death will occur quickly. To keep the blood pH within its proper range, the body will take either alkaline or acid ions from other areas of the body, including the saliva, urine, bone, and even the cells. When the body develops an overly acid condition, the organs and cells gradually become acidic even though the blood pH may appear to be within the normal range. The blood pH is the last pH indicator to drop because it steals the substances needed to maintain its pH from the rest of the body, and by time the blood pH drop occurs, death is near. If the blood pH is even close to the bottom end of the normal range it is time to take serious action. Doctors rarely pay any attention to the pH factor and if the blood pH is within the range of 7.25 to 7.40, then they think that all is well. They fail to consider that while a blood pH below 7.25 means almost instantaneous death, a blood pH of below 7.30 can mean close to death or a slow death. Yes, you can still be alive with a blood pH of 7.27 but that does not mean that you are healthy. The one very powerful reason that blood pH is so critical is because of the immune system. The immune system functions best at a pH of 7.35, not lower, not higher. For this one reason, it is neglect on the part of the medical profession to ignore one of the most important indicators of health. Another reason that pH is important is the regulation of geAcid-

Alkaline pH balance and Cancerne expression by proteins known as histones. The way that they bind to DNA is very sensitive to pH.

For these reasons and others, it is very important to monitor both your urine pH and your saliva pH. For an individual, the easiest method to monitor is the pH reading observed when the urine is checked when first rising in the morning, before eating , drinking, or exercising. The reason for this is that the urine pH can change very quickly after either eating, drinking, or exercise. Testing the urine pH is good as it can be done daily or even more frequently and because it is a good indicator of how much acid or alkali that the body has to eliminate in order to maintain balance. The urine pH can range from less than 6.0 to almost 8.0 depending on health and when the pH is measured. This reading is affected by the amount of water ingested, the types and amounts of foods last eaten, the amount of carbon dioxide present from exercise, any lactic acid present from cancers, and the bodies buffering ability which is a factor of the bodies mineral content. Ideally, the early morning urine pH should be near or slightly above 7.0. Do not eat, drink, or exercise before checking this pH reading. When cancer is present, this reading will often be near or below 6.0. A reading this low does not mean that you have cancer however, it may mean that you are at higher than normal risk of developing cancer.. I repeat here that the significance of urine pH is that this is an indication of how much acid or base that your body needs to eliminate to keep the blood pH from getting out of range. The blood pH is more stable and is a more reliable indication of critical health conditions. A normal blood pH is about 7.25 to 7.40 with 7.35 being ideal, but taking a blood sample is required. It is important here to bring out the importance of ideal or optimum. The ideal level or optimum level of anything is the level at which your entire body operates most efficiently. Saliva pH can range from 6.0 to 7.8 with 7.0 being ideal. Saliva pH can also be tested frequently but it is less important as an indicator except when it gets below pH 6.7. The reason for this is that the saliva is designed to be alkaline for digestion purposes. If it is frequently acid, this means that the salivary glands are not able to extract enough alkalinity from the blood which most likely means that the blood pH is lower than it should be. It is also a strong indication that other organs are not receiving enough alkalinity and may be reducing their functionality. When the pH is too low, the pancreas suffers and pancreatin production is reduced. As you will read later, pancreatin is important for fighting cancer.

Medical professionals and researchers often ignore pH as an important clue although many are aware that the pH drop is associated with health problems. One doctor from Italy decided to test the idea of pH vs cancer and found that by raising the blood pH with Sodium bicarbonate, the cancer tended to disappear. He now treats cancer with Sodium bicarbonate. While it is not clear whether low pH is a result of cancer or if cancer is a result of low pH, it is important to know that fixing the acid pH condition cannot hurt and will likely improve chances of recovery and survival. It is also important to understand that pH influences important biological processes such as genetic regulation, enzyme activity, and protein production. The closer to pH 7.35 that your blood is, the better your enzymes, hormones, and cellular functions will work. Standard blood testing does not even bother to monitor the blood pH. This should be a standard part of the test as it is a valuable indicator. While normal blood pH is 7.25 to 7.40, I would be concerned at any time that the pH approaches either extreme. If your blood pH is below 7.29, this is probably a good indicator that something is not right. The fact is that your body has an optimum pH and that every function of the body is at its best or near its best at this pH. The kidneys function better, the pancreas functions better, the liver functions better, the immune system functions better, hormones and enzymes function better, and even the genetic control of the cells functions better at this optimum pH. Perhaps this might be a hint as to why we do get cancer and to why modern medicine can not cure it.

A major issue that appears to be a problem with low blood pH is one of bone depletion. When the body looses its ability to properly buffer the blood pH, it starts using bone for this purpose, causing osteoporosis. This is not the only cause of osteoporosis, but it can and does occur. The same conditions can cause dental decay. The depletion of calcium from the body should not be taken lightly. It is very important in the development of cancer. Cancer cells are often deficient of calcium compared to normal cells. It is also interesting to note that one of the most painful parts of cancer is when it metastasizes to the bone. It does this because the bone has lost much of its alkalinity and had porous areas where the cancer can invade.

The regulation of pH is also important to a major part of the genetic control system is a group of proteins referred to as histones, which bind to DNA and may act to repress the action of specific genes. These proteins are sensitive to pH as well as other physiological changes. It is known that an acid pH condition will change the shape of proteins and affect their binding properties. It is very likely that acidity within a cell will cause certain histones to release their associated genes for processing. If the affected histone is one that controls replication, cancer is the likely outcome.

It is also well documented that many of the things associated with cancer, including tobacco smoke, carbonated drinks including diet drinks with artificial sweeteners, artificial sweeteners, high meat consumption, high sugar intake, and diets low in vegetable material, will lower the pH and cause acidic conditions in the body. It is also documented that many things associated with decreasing cancer also cause the body to become more alkaline such as drinking green tea and eating lots of fresh raw vegetables and fruits. Actually, while it does not always work entirely on its own, the best-documented cause of spontaneous remission of cancer is a diet of fresh raw fruits and vegetables. This does not mean that vegetarians never get cancer but it is true that they do have a far lower incidence of cancer. A lot depends on the specific vegetables and fruits eaten as not all fruits and vegetable are alkalizing. One noticeable condition exists though; a person with a normally alkaline pH condition will almost never have cancer.

An acid pH condition within a cell may also affect the respiration activities within a cell. This may cause a condition that is present in cancer sufferers which is higher than normal amounts of lactic acid. The body normally uses aerobic respiration, in which the cell's mitochondria uses glucose and oxygen to produce energy and carbon dioxide, a very efficient metabolism. The carbon dioxide is then normally carried away by the blood and eliminated from the body through breathing. Cancer cells generally use anaerobic respiration and produce lactic acid as a product of cellular respiration rather than carbon dioxide and the mitochondria are less functional. Since the body cannot exhale the lactic acid, the liver metabolizes it and converts it to glycogen. Glycogen is how the body stores energy and when energy is needed, glycogen is split into glucose. This is convenient for the cancer because it needs large amounts of glucose for continued growth. This places the body into a cycle of continuously feeding the cancer and at the same time making the body more acidic which encourages additional cancer growth. Note that any ingested sugar or foods with a high glycemic index (those foods that require a large amount of insulin to be released or high sugar content) will be converted to glycogen and will also support the growth of cancer. If you have significant cancerous growth in your body and a blood glucose test is performed after a 12 hour fast, the blood glucose will register below normal, often well below. This is in itself a strong indication that cancer thrives off of glucose and that reducing glycemic intake will help fight cancer. The opposite end of the glucose tolerance spectrum is a high blood glucose level after 12 hours of fasting. In this case, the body itself has become resistant to the presence of insulin and is referred to as insulin resistance. It should be noted here that insulin resistance can increase the risk of cancer as well as the chances of many other illnesses. This also brings into focus another aspect of cancer, the fact that it metabolizes glucose and the cancer cell membrane is designed to import large amounts of glucose, then it will also import many glycogen based molecules.

This is one aspect that chemotherapy does try to take advantage of. Attach a poison to glucose and the cancer cells will absorb more of it than normal cells, at least in theory. This is also a part of how some natural substances such as cyanogenic glycosides can attack cancers without harming normal cells.

Insulin resistance can cause additional problems inside of the cells. Insulin is not just a factor for the regulation of sugar, it is a hormone, a communication molecule that may be secreted by cells in one area of the body that causes cells in another area to preform certain functions. Insulin can also influence several functions such as growth, cellular respiration, electron transport, and even immunity. It is the electron transport process that takes place in the mitochondria that produces the necessary energy for each cell to maintain its processes. When the conversion of glucose to carbon dioxide takes place, energy is extracted with maximum efficiency and is transported through the electron transport system of the mitochondria. When this process fails to be carried through to completion, the end product is lactic acid, which is carried by the blood stream back to the liver, where it is recycled back to glucose and glycogen.

There are drugs such as hydrazine sulfate available to reduce the lactic acid metabolism by the liver and many cancer sufferers have successfully used them. There are claims that Dichloroacetate (DCA) appears to reactivate the mitochondria, allowing normal cellular respiration to resume. Unfortunately, the FDA is blocking the sale of some of these drugs in the US although they are accepted in many other countries. Many long-term cancer survivors swear by these drugs and there appear to be few side effects associated with them. If hydrazine sulfate is considered, the user should be cautious, as it is a MAOI and can interfere with other drugs. Other drugs are available to reduce the transport of needed nutrients such as glycogen or glucose into the cancer cell. These drugs have a positive benefit but unless proper pH is restored, cancer is not likely to be stopped.

There are also numerous other nutritional substances that help with the conversion of glucose to carbon dioxide. One of these is Niacin, (nicotinic acid) which is used to form NAD and NADH, both of which are critical to the process. It appears that vitamin B3 is important but there is also significant information that the nicotinic acid form is far more effective than the commonly available niacinamide form of B3. Vitamin D3 (cholecalciferol) is another substance that works not only to aid certain processes, but is also used as a hormone, intended to signal certain cells to preform certain functions. Vitamin D3, however, goes way beyond this and is of major importance, not only to immunity, but also in regulation of genes and gene expression. Vitamin D3 is crucial to the maintenance of Calcium in almost all cells in the body as well as to maintain the pH. The point is really that to resist cancer and to fight cancer, the body needs the proper amounts as well as the proper forms of nutrition, enzymes, co-enzymes, and hormones. Again, cancer, as well as any health problem is the result of the weakest link. Among the most important of all of these enzymes and hormones is insulin.

Insulin also plays an important part of this process of anaerobic metabolism. Cancer cells often have many times more insulin receptors on their membranes than normal cells do. This allows the cancer cells to absorb more glucose than normal cells. Some anti-cancer drugs may utilize this factor by attaching a glucose molecule to the active product (gluconate, glycosides) to increase absorption into cancer cells. Additionally, some therapies use insulin to increase the transfer of anticancer substances into tumor cells. This process is referred to as insulin potentiation. Some natural therapies utilize these same processes and characteristics. It should be noted here that being diabetic is a serious risk factor for many cancers.

Another of the most observable physiological conditions of many but not all cancer patients is anemia. Insufficient red blood cells increase cancerous growth and will deprive normal cells of the oxygen needed to fight cancer. Cancer appears to have an affinity for iron. If a person has serious cancer growth it is important to augment the blood supply of red blood cells, hemoglobin, and hematocrit, if they are very low. Ferritin iron in the blood should be kept below 100. Vitamin and mineral supplementation often helps and should be used first but drugs such as Procrit may be required in some cases. Changes in white blood cell counts may also occur, especially with chemotherapy. Any change in the white blood cells, especially any reduction, should be considered critical.

Another change that occurs when cancer is present is that there is a change in the amounts of various amino acids that are present. Amino acids are building blocks of the body and are specifically combined to form proteins that may function as enzymes, hormones, or precursors for other proteins. The presence of certain amino acids is significantly reduced in many cases and other amino acids may increase. Amino acid levels may be checked with a blood test. Some amino acids may be adjusted by adding or removing certain foods from the diet. Others require additional changes such as amino acid supplements to adjust their levels. It has been shown that pH selectively affects the control of various amino acids and the proteins that they are incorporated into. Both cysteine and methionine are essential amino acids that are critical to good health because they are highly utilized in the body. One example of an amino acid in cancer is cysteine which is a precursor to glutathione. In one extensive study, higher plasma total cysteine concentrations were significantly associated with a lower risk of breast cancer. For women in the highest quintile of plasma total cysteine, compared with those in the lowest quintile, the relative risk was 0.44. This is an incredibly strong indication that cysteine is extremely important in both avoiding cancer as well as in fighting it. In other studies, it is shown that deficiencies of the main dietary sources of methyl donors, methionine and choline, lead to the formation of liver cancer in rodents.

Hormones

Some of these proteins are hormones and one thing important to know about cancer is that various cancers may influence hormone levels in the body while most cancers rely on the presence of certain hormones. Examples of hormone sensitive cancers may be breast, ovarian, prostate, and endometrial cancers. Not all forms of these cancers are hormone sensitive, however. Hormones are proteins that modulate or influence the action of other proteins or cellular functions. The blood can also be tested for the levels of these hormones and therapy can be administered to correct for some imbalances that may be found. Some important examples of cancer related hormones are VEGF (vascular epithelial growth factor) and CEA (Carcinoembryonic antigen). Certain drugs that reduce hormones are used to help fight cancer and while they may have benefits, the cancer will not be completely eliminated until the conditions that foster cancer are eliminated.

As a note: There is one hormone in particular that forms the basis of many of the body's hormones and DHEA is the one to remember. While it is the base hormone that many of the sex hormones are built on, it is also a very important immunity booster. Many people with cancer, when tested are found to be very deficient in DHEA. While there are studies that DHEA can accelerate cancer growth "in vitro" (in the test tube or culture dish), there has not been sufficient study to determine whether increased DHEA levels might improve immunity enough to offset the acceleration of cancer growth. See: Dihydroepiandosterone

Other proteins are combined to form enzymes and co-enzymes. Enzymes are special proteins that enable or assist specific chemical reactions to take place. Some enzymes such as the COX-2 (cyclooxygenase-2) enzyme are common to many cancers and the use of specific inhibitors may help fight these cancers. Other enzymes that are necessary for normal cell function may not be present in sufficient quantities. Increasing these enzymes with supplements can also be beneficial in fighting cancer. One important example is pancreatin (pancreatic enzyme). A co-enzyme is protein that assists other enzymes with performing their functions. Some of these co-enzymes may also be present in reduced quantities and require supplementation. Cancer sufferers may often need and should receive co-enzyme-Q10 supplements.

There are some health professionals who believe that the presence of parasites in the body can cause, aggravate, or accelerate cancer. Little research has been done to support or disprove this, however there is some supporting evidence, which should not be ignored by the medical profession. The problem with parasites is that they steal important nutrition, dump their wastes into the body, and excrete hormones that may increase cancerous growth or impede immunity. Parasites also serve as a distraction for NK cells that are responsible for killing cancer cells and suppress the immune system. Some parasites have been positively linked with cancer and for this reason; cancer patients should be screened for parasite protein markers using a blood test. Stool tests and such are very unreliable and should not be completely relied on, especially since not all parasites are intestinal. Also, it is not reliable to use eosinophil levels as the only indicator as many parasites are able to suppress these white blood cells. Among these cancer related parasites are Candida albicans, several types of worms, and several virus forms. Eliminating these parasites with herbals and a device called the "zapper" may help and rarely causes any problems and these problems are minor. There are also traditional medicine treatments for parasites but these may be harsh and may cause additional problems.

Toxins and waste

There are other therapists who feel that the body may be loaded with toxins and wastes accumulated in the bowels and other organs. There are herbals and cleanses that can help remove these unwanted byproducts of living. These liver cleanses, kidney flushes, and colon cleanses are generally harmless if done correctly and have definite health benefits. The result of cleanses and flushes are often immediate and obvious and for this reason, they are highly recommended. There are many different types of flushes, enemas, and cleanses so it is up to the user to choose their path. A good choice is to visit a couple of colonic therapy spas and discuss their options and suggestions. These flushes and cleanses have been popular for years and have been used without negative indications or problems. While many doctors feel that they are not proven, they generally do not cause harm and may actually help.

Nutrition

Probably the most important alternative to conventional therapy is good general nutritional support. This means both eating the right things at the right time and not eating at the right times. Improper nutrition is behind many health problems including cancer. Many people with cancer are "midnight snackers, over-weight, diabetic, tobacco smokers, etc). These are serious problematic habits that encourage cancer growth.

Otherwise, certain vitamins and other antioxidants have been shown to reduce the chance of having cancer as well as being very helpful in defeating it. A person who is actually in good nutritional condition (not appearing to be in good condition) rarely gets cancer and has a much better chance of surviving cancer as well as surviving the harsh treatment offered by conventional therapies. Cancer sufferers may often benefit from using as much as 10 to 20 times the normal amounts of specific required vitamins. There are some clinical tests that have shown that certain vitamins do not help. These tests should be viewed with caution as the protocol usually includes only a single vitamin supplement or uses these vitamins at or below minimal levels of effectiveness. Several recent studies have presented the idea that supplements do not help. These studies are often flawed and biased. They do show that vitamins bought off of the store shelf are not of much benefit and this is for several reasons, including poor quality, poor absorption, incorrect form of the vitamins, and minimal amounts rather than optimal. Good nutrition means having sufficient amounts of the proper form of all necessary vitamins and minerals to insure proper metabolism. Any vitamin or mineral that is not present at the required levels will tend to skew the results. Any vitamin or mineral in the wrong form will skew results. An excellent example is vitamin B3 which comes in 2 main forms, Niacin (which causes a flush) and niacinamide. Both have some benefits but in some studies, the real Niacin (full flush) has far better benefits in most cases although some people can not handle it. Another good example is vitamin B12 which is available in 3 forms, the good form, methylcobalamin which can cross the blood brain barrier, hydroxycobalamin, and the cheaper common form cyanocobalamin which requires a long, energy draining process to be converted to methylcobalamin.

Remember that it is the weakest link in the chain that will break. It is important that high quality vitamins of the right form be used, as many vitamins offered through standard stores may not be of the best quality. My recommendation is to skip the drug store shelf brands and go for the better vitamins. The absolute best source of vitamins is from high quality foods but sadly, when your health is down, you need serious help. Also, it should be noted that the vitamins provided in some hospitals might be among the worst as some patients have reported expelling entire undigested pills in their stool. It has been shown that only certain mega-dose vitamins can extend life expectancy in terminal cases by as much as 4 times or more and can significantly reduce recurrences of many cancers. One thing to note is that if you take a vitamin supplement, mineral supplement, or some form of anti-oxidant and you notice a boost in energy or some other improvement the first couple of times, this is a definite indication of some deficiency and you should continue this supplementation.

The RDA or recommended daily allowance of a supplement is basically the amount of that substance that is added to the diet will avoid extreme nutritional disorders from showing up. It does not prevent obscure or long term problems from manifesting. An example of this is Vitamin C, which leads to scurvy if a person does not get enough. While the RDA will prevent major symptoms of scurvy from appearing, minor symptoms such as small cracks and fissures in blood vessels may still appear. These can lead to hardening of the arteries and eventually heart attacks. Note that the body uses cholesterol to patch these cracks in the arteries and capillaries. This is why some medical professionals mistakenly believe that cholesterol is the problem, even though the statin drugs that they prescribe do not significantly reduce atherosclerosis or heart attacks .

It is often suggested that care must be used when taking vitamins at therapeutic levels as excessive amounts of some vitamins can cause additional health problems. This concern is particularly true of fat-soluble vitamins such as A, D, E, and K. This should also be carefully considered. For example, the RDA of vitamin D is 400 IU daily but while exposed to bright sunlight, the body can manufacture up to 3 million IU of vitamin D per day according to some sources! It is obvious that something is wrong with the RDA rating for vitamin D. In response to this, the value was raised to paltry 600 IU daily. Vitamin D is particularly important for individuals with cancer as it aids in the transport of calcium into the body and to cells. Many cancer patients benefit from taking 5000 IU daily to 10,000 daily or more. Use caution and taking more than 2800 IU per day should be done under a doctor's advice. Very few foods provide any significant amounts of vitamin D.

The RDA for vitamin A is 5000 IU per day. On this basis you should not eat spinach, sweet potatoes, or most peppers as all of these exceed this amount of vitamin A per serving. A serving of beef liver can supply 75000 IU of Vitamin A. A serving of carrots can contain 19000 IU of the same. Again, something is wrong with the RDA rating for vitamin A. Vitamin A is important but it should come from natural sources whenever possible. There are also several forms and the form taken is important. Retinol is a form of vitamin A that comes from many meats and animal products. Carotenoids come from plant sources and are generally considered to be better. You should also know that Retinol will actually block the absorption of vitamin D.

There are actually 7 main forms of vitamin E and all are important while the standard off the shelf form of vitamin E only contains one of these, alpha tocopherol which is the cheapest and easiest to make. Even then, it is usually in the form of alpha tocopherol acetate. However, the gamma tocopherol is likely the most important form. Among the functions of vitamin is as an antioxidant.

There is also a vitamin K1 and a vitamin K2 and both are important.

It is very difficult to overdose on the water-soluble vitamins such as Vitamin C or the B vitamins as the body will readily excrete any excesses. There is a limitation as to how much and how quickly the body can excrete these however, so caution should be used. The intake of most vitamins should be spread out over the entire day rather than being taken all at once. Many vitamins should be taken with meals as this improves absorption. Vitamin C is best taken with a juice that normally contains vitamin C, such as orange juice or grapefruit juice. Always avoid drinks that contain corn sweeteners, high amounts of sugars, artificial sweeteners, etc. Read the labels of what you drink or eat.

It is most important to remove the negative nutritional influences such as excessive refined sugars, carbonated drinks, artificial sweeteners, alcohol, fermented yeast products, and excessive fats from the diet. Especially important is the elimination of refined white sugar as this is literally cancer food. It is very important to eliminate excesses of animal protein and foods with a high glycemic index from the diet. Processed foods often have hidden sugars and other chemicals that will support cancer growth. Avoid all processed foods if possible. Avoid hydrogenated oils and fatty foods. These negative nutritional influences are the main source of acidic pH that is associated with cancer and may be the root cause of cancer.

Herbals

Some herbals and supplements are reputed to have very positive benefits when fighting cancer. Among these supplements are Essiac tea, Paw Paw extract, Curcumin, apricot pits, shark liver oil, modified citrus pectin (MCP), Feverfew, Ginger, Resveratrol, Genestein, Kefir, Methylsulfonylmethionine (MSM), green tea, carotenoids, and phytonutrients as well as many others. Most of these herbals are harmless but care should be used as some herbals may interfere with each other as well as interfering with traditional medications that may be used. Some of the effects of these herbal supplements may vary from COX-2 inhibitors to pH regulation, prevention of lactic acid metabolism, reduction of metastases, reduction of vascularization, and provision of needed nutrients. Other supplements such as Melatonin offer benefits such as improved sleep, improved immune function, and reduction of anemia. Whatever supplements you may use the quality and source of the supplement is important. Many supplements are unregulated and as a result, there can be a wide variation in quality.

When you ask most oncologists, they may tell you that there are not any clinical tests to show that the natural therapies mentioned above work. This is not true; there have been numerous tests to show that many of these alternatives provide beneficial results. Possibly the oncologist may not be interested in looking or may just not be aware. Otherwise, there are not any valid tests that show that they do not work either, otherwise, they would be quick to point these out. In fact, they will dig hard to find anything negative about any alternative or natural therapy. Even when tests exist to show that something does not work, these tests should be viewed carefully as they may often be biased in order to provide the appearance of ineffectiveness. This is often achieved by using a dosage that is below the minimum effective dose or by allowing the control group to use some other substance that is just as effective. Remember that the use of nutrition and supplements competes with the medical industry for your money. The truth is that you are likely to receive far more benefit than harm from a properly designed therapeutic nutritional support plan. After all, the best way to beat cancer is to be healthy. Good nutrition does not cause you to get nausea, vomit, lose weight, or make your hair fall out. Good nutrition does not cause your cancer to return or to spread.

Steps to defeating Cancer

So, what does one need to do in order to have the greatest success when fighting cancer?

Boost the natural immune system and its normal function.

In the long run, it is the immune system that will beat cancer. Take supplements and eat foods that will help the immune system and improve general immune system health. Avoid therapies that damage the immune system in any way. Get plenty of restful sleep, as this is when the immune system docs the most effective repair. Taking melatonin significantly improves sleep and boosts the immune system. Taking the right supplements can boost your immune function and help you feel better. Ask your doctor to monitor your blood for immune factors such as blood cell counts, tumor markers, and other health indicators such as blood pH.

Restore the body's pH balance.

Cancer will not be completely defeated until normal pH is restored.

The best way to achieve this is through eating fresh natural raw fruits and vegetables, especially those reputed to alkalize the body such as lemon and grapefruit. One of the best ways to achieve pH balance is by juicing dark green vegetables such as broccoli, spinach, and kale. Lemons and grapefruit are very alkalizing citrus fruits. Fresh vegetable juice and tomato juices are also beneficial but carrots, noni, and other vegetables with high sugar content should not be overused. Canned vegetable juices have been heated or cooked and will not have many of the preferred enzymes which are destroyed by heat. Frozen vegetables will have some of the enzymes still active but not necessarily all. Frozen vegetables should have close to the same alkalizing value as fresh vegetables. Freshly sprouted vegetables contain many beneficial enzymes that are easily absorbed when juiced. Among the most popular are broccoli sprouts, wheat grass sprouts, and barley sprouts.

If the cancer is to a critical point, some people may choose to use cesium or rubidium salts. These can have a dramatic effect when used but can cause serious problems if not used correctly. It may also be beneficial to drink an alkaline mineral water with Calcium, Magnesium, Potassium and other mineral salts in it such as sodium bicarbonate. Ask your doctor to monitor your blood pH, calcium, magnesium, iron, and potassium levels, and keep you advised. It is important to repeat, the medical profession feels that the normal range of blood pH is 7.25 to 7.40, it is absolutely important to carefully move close to 7.35. It may not only help you but may help your doctor learn something new.

Restore the blood to normal function.

Cancer patients with anemia or near anemic conditions are the least likely to survive. Since blood carries oxygen to the cells and since anemia reduces the oxygen carrying capacity of the blood, cancer becomes almost impossible to beat. For this reason, it is imperative to bring the blood into balance. To accomplish this, it is necessary to have the proper amount of iron available to make hemoglobin. The ferritin iron level should be below 100 while keeping hemoglobin and hemocritin up. Melatonin is very important in reducing anemia and has many other benefits as well. Melatonin should be taken at night, usually just before bed. Normal dosage is from 3 to 12 mg but many cancer sufferers take up to 20 mg or more without problems. It is actually possible to take as much as 70 mg daily as some tests have shown. Do not over do it, however. Take enough to allow a good night's sleep. It is also better to take a little and then more later if needed. Vitamin B12 also helps reduce anemia along with Folic acid but again, take the proper form. The best form of vitamin B12 is methylcobalamin but almost all B12 found in stores is cyanocobalamin. Some cancers reportedly use folic acid so those large amounts may need to be avoided only with these cancers. DHA from fish oil has some positive benefits in reducing anemia. Cod liver oil has been known for its health boosting power for many years. When the above supplements fail to reduce the anemia, drugs such as Procrit may be called for, but this should always be combined with iron supplements and only as a last resort. Daily supplementation with shark liver oil will boost platelet production if needed. Uncooked leeks, spinach, apricots, and raisins are helpful in providing iron for the blood. Vitamin C assists in the absorption of iron while zinc and vitamin E will interfere, so they should not be taken at the same time. Coffee and tea interfere with iron absorption. Vitamin B12 is important and as a supplement, methylcobalamin is probably the best source. As a food, liver is a good source of blood building vitamins.

Avoid things that cause harm to your body.

While your doctor may have you sign consent forms and just offer that it is routine, some of the tests and therapies that they provide are seriously damaging. Whenever possible, avoid PET scans, Cat scans, and any other procedure that exposes your body to excess radiation. Even mammograms are highly damaging. Biopsies allow cancer to spread faster and further.

Stop the cancer from spreading further.

Using certain natural supplements will cause cancer cells to stick together and keep them from migrating to other areas of the body. Supplements such as MCP (modified citrus pectin) have been shown to bind cancer cells to each other and to neighboring cells thereby reducing the chance of metastases spreading. Curcumin and catechin have been shown to inhibit metastasis. Proteolytic enzymes attack the protein layers on the surface of cancer cells which prevents them from binding and in turn this helps stop metastasis.

Remove cancers nutritional sources.

Cancers thrive on sugars and other foods with a high glycemic index. Avoid these as much as possible. This includes avoiding starches such as wheat and potatoes. Avoid sugar alcohols such as artificial sweeteners. Excessive iron in the blood supports cancer growth. Fructose and high fructose corn syrup cause fatty liver which increases health problems. One of the fastest and most effective ways of shrinking a tumor is a water fast. Nothing but pure clean water for 24 hours.

Cleanse the body to remove unwanted toxins and unnecessary substances such as fat. This includes fasting (not taking in any nutrition except good clean pure water) which in itself can help defeat cancer. Some of the most effective alternative therapies include fasting as a part of their regime. It may also be an odd artifact of chemotherapy that occasionally allows it to be of some benefit. Many chemotherapy patients are very sick as a result of their treatment, cannot keep food down, and loose weight. It is known that when the body does not receive sufficient nutrition as in a fasting condition, it will turn against various cells within the body causing the immune system to attack the most abnormal and least efficient cells present. As a result, the body will increase its efforts to kill cancer cells. Also, during fasting, the demands that are placed on the excretory organs are reduced allowing the body to concentrate on removing substances that it might normally be able to during periods of normal activity. These are often substances that might be more difficult to excrete such as lead and mercury. On of the groups that have the lowest rate of cancer in the U.S. Is the Mormons. It is a Mormon tradition to fast at least one day every month. They are also much stricter about eating a natural, wholesome, healthy diet.

Restrain or eliminate the hormones and enzymes that support cancer growth.

There are numerous natural supplements available such as Feverfew, ginger, goldenseal, and green tea, which contain constituents that will inhibit the COX-2 enzyme and others. Curcumin directly inhibits COX-2 and also inhibits angiogenic growth in tumors thereby reducing the blood supply.

Oxygenate and remove carbon dioxide.

Cancer does not like oxygen and carbon dioxide helps keep the cancers environment acid. As stated above, it is important to reduce or eliminate any anemic condition. It is also important to get plenty of exercise, outdoors fresh air, and plenty of sunlight. Statistics show that cancer sufferers who get plenty of exercise, outdoor air, and sunlight generally live twice as long or even longer than those who do not.

Check your attitude.

Having a good attitude is important in fighting cancer. Attitude is your **perception** of how things are. Laugh and have a good time rather than being despondent and depressed. Laughter helps oxygenate your blood, causes the production of chemical agents that aid in healing, reduces stress, and helps with recovery. Also, get lots of fresh air, sunshine, and blue sky whenever possible. Ask your self what you want your life to be. Listen to your favorite music, do the things that you have always wanted to do. Reach out to others, being alone does not help. These things will at least double the life expectancy of the cancer sufferer and if nothing else make the remaining time here more enjoyable. If there are things about your life, family, or friends that have bothered you, now is the time to resolve them. If you have problems that are eating at you emotionally, you can not devote a full effort to eliminating cancer. Belief, vision, and ethic are all, important aspects of attitude. You must believe that you can achieve the goal of being cancer free. It happens all the time. There are numerous documented cases of spontaneous remission of cancers, even in cases where the person was death bed terminal. There are cases where cancer sufferers arose from a coma to walk away, cancer free. It is also important to be able to see the possibility of a long productive life ahead, to have a vision of success in beating cancer. But belief and vision alone are not going to produce results. The fulfillment of the vision often comes with effort on your part. A work ethic is required. You must follow whatever diet or program you choose. You must maintain your attitude in order to succeed. There may be times when conditions appear to worsen, keep to your program.

Remarkable recovery

There many unexplained recoveries from terminal cancer that have occurred over the years that many doctors are not even aware of. People were sent home to die and who showed up, sometimes years later, completely cancer free even though their surgical wounds and other signs were still visible. These patients suffered from all kinds of cancers, including melanoma, stomach, liver, lung, and pancreatic cancer. In the book "Remarkable Recovery" there only appeared one common connection between all of the subjects. There seemed to be a common link that all of the individuals who recovered had felt an electrical surge through their body before the cancer went away.

Could electricity offer a solution?

Supplements from various sources and benefits

Acetaminophen

works not only as an analgesic, it increases the effectiveness of some other NSAIDs and of some opiates. It should be noted however, that acetaminophen can cause liver damage, especially when glutathione levels are low. It is actually a leading cause of liver and kidney damage in western society. Acetaminophen can reduce niacin, thiamin, and pyridoxine in the liver, which are important vitamins. It can also be oxidized to a toxic substance that reduces glutathione, which can cause the death of liver cells. Once the liver cells start dying, kidney cells soon follow. The risk of liver damage increases when combined with alcohol or other substances that may cause liver damage. NAC (n-acetyl cysteine) can be given to help reduce this problem as it promotes the production of glutathione and is used as an antidote. Alpha Lipoic acid is also beneficial as an antioxidant. Vitamin E and melatonin are also beneficial, as is silymarin (the active ingredient in Milk Thistle). Acetaminophen is the main ingredient in Tylenol and Panadol and is also in Hydrocodone, Sudafed, and Theraflu. While doctors may disregard this, I feel that it is recommended to avoid acetaminophen when fighting cancer to avoid additional health consequences. When fighting cancer, the health of the liver becomes critically important.

Alcohol

consumption is a definite risk factor in several cancers, including head and neck cancers, oral cancer, esophageal cancer, breast cancer, testicular cancer, liver cancer, and especially pancreatic cancer. There is some reduction of risk for lymphoma (both Hodgkin's and non-Hodgkin's) when small amounts are consumed. Liver damage seems to significantly contribute to cancer mortality. Supplements that are beneficial in counteracting the effects of alcohol are NAC (n-acetyl Cysteine), ALA (alpha lipoic acid), and milk thistle.

Aloe Immune

is a refined extract of aloe vera that has certain constituents concentrated, including acemannan, glyco-polymannans, and aloe polymannans. These particular substances are reputedly responsible for increased immune system activity and the activation of macrophages.*Aloe vera* juice provides strong support to the immune system and is well known for its healing properties. It is important in activating NK cells. Additionally, it contains several alkalizing minerals that are important in fighting cancer. It also contains several cancer fighting vitamins and may contain a number of other anticancer nutrients as well. Among these nutrients are emodin, mannose, and lectin, all of which have been shown to have anti-tumor effects. It also supplies amylase enzymes that assist pancreatin in attacking cancer cells. The use of aloe vera has been shown in studies to increase the effectiveness of certain cancer treatments such as with the chemotherapy agents cyclophosphamide (Cytoxan, Neosar) and 5-fluorouracil (5-FU). An extract of aloe vera, Emodin, inhibited cell proliferation and induced apoptosis in human liver cancer cell lines through both p53- and p21-dependent pathways Emodin also blocks the growth of some head and neck cancer cells in vitro. Another study suggests that Aloe vera consumption can reduce the risk of lung cancer. Other studies show that some components of aloe, such as acemannan, aloeride, and di(2-ethylhexyl)phthalate (DEHP) may have immunomodulating and anticancer effects

Alpha-Lipoic acid (ALA)

is an antioxidant, gene expression regulator, and it helps regenerate other antioxidants. It can independently extend life expectancy by as much as 25%. It has` also been shown to help regenerate failed livers and other organs. Suggested usage is 300 to 1500 mg daily and I have not found any studies indicating that these levels would not be safe. ALA helps regenerate vitamin C and E as well as several other antioxidants such as glutathione and CoQ10. An important point to note about ALA is that it increases the glucose uptake of normal cells and reduces insulin resistance. *It is not known whether or not it will increase the glucose uptake by cancerous cells. It does lower blood glucose levels and therefore may reduce the glucose available to cancerous cells but this has not been documented.* ALA has been combined with high dose vitamin C therapy and this combination has produced very good results but oncologists are trying to stop this because it does not make money. Another valuable therapy is LDN (low dose naltrexone) with ALA, which has also shown amazing results, including a cure of a patient with pancreatic cancer..

Alpha-linolenic acid

is a precursor omega-3 fatty acid, which can be converted by the body to EPA and DHA. All three have definite anti-cancer benefits. This is combined with cottage cheese as part of the Budwig cancer diet. Flaxseed is high in Alpha-linolenic acid.

L-Arginine

Increases levels of white blood cells but may accelerate some cancers. L-Arginine is considered to be a conditionally essential amino acid in that the body will normally produce a sufficient amount but under stress, it may need supplementation. It is a precursor in the production of several important compounds and is considered important in immune function. In some cancers, such as breast cancer, **L-Arginine has been shown to increase NK cells as well as other immune cells**. In some cases, L-Arginine may nearly double NK cell activity. L-Arginine should be used with caution in those experiencing renal or kidney failures. Normally, up to 14 grams of L-Arginine can be taken daily without complications. As much as 30 gm. per day may be taken but may produce side effects such as nausea and diarrhea.

Ambrotose

is a supplement composed of eight essential glyconutrients. These glyconutrients are mannose, galactose, fucose, glucose, xylose, nacetylgalactosamine, n-acetylglucosamine, and n-acetylneuramic acid. It is felt that these essential glyconutrients are important for overall health. The uses of this product for treating cancer is suspect as the sugars may actually feed cancer. I could not find any relevant scientific studies supporting the use of Ambrotose or similar supplements to treat cancer.

Amygdalin

In a study using beagle dogs, the dogs (4 animals/sex/group) were administered 500 mg amygdalin in 10 ml solution respectively, intravenously and orally after overnight fast. Blood was sampled from jugular vein and urine was collected by a funnel. Faeces were removed from the funnel. The major part of the dose (71%) was recovered in the urines collected during 6 h following intravenous amygdalin administration. The fraction of the dose excreted by glomerular filtration was calculated using the ratio of diatrizoate (which was administered simultaneously) clearance to amygdalin clearance, showing that 97% of the amount of amygdalin to be expected was recovered from the urine. The result of the experiments after intravenous administration were analyzed assuming a two-compartment model. No prunasin, which is an indicator of cyanogenic toxicity, was detected in urine. After oral administration of amygdalin a very low maximal plasma level is found after approximately 0.75 h. Only 2.3% of the amygdalin was systematically available. Prunasin was found in plasma and urine of the dogs. In the urine collected during 6 h following amygdalin administration only about 1% of the dose was recovered unchanged and 21% of the dose was identified as prunasin. In humans, pharmacological studies have shown that amygdalin is broken down to HCN, benzaldehyde and glucose by enzymes found in gut bacteria, but not intracellularly in humans, however, it is claimed that it does enter cancer cells, causing apoptosis. Animal and human tissues contain no significant concentrations of ß-glucosidase, the only known activating enzyme of hydrolysis of cyanogenic glycosides in vivo.

Reports of Acute toxicity studies in humans

From 1 to 10 g of amygdalin have been given parenterally (not through the digestive tract) in humans, without acute toxicity. This indirectly suggests that there is no significant metabolism of the intact injected glycoside which is consistent with the absence of ß-glucosidase. The cyanide-containing breakdown products have well-defined toxicities, and 50 mg of hydrogen cyanide can be fatal. In the case of oral dosing of amygdalin, a toxic potential is present. Intestinal flora produce ß-glucosidase in the gastrointestinal lumen. It was reported that **oral laetrile (amygdalin) could be 40 times more toxic than parenterally administered doses**. This is likely due to the free HCN released by the ß-glucosidase enzyme produced in the gut. The reported lethal dose of amygdalin for man when ingested is reported to be in the range of 0.02-0.13 mmol/kg bw. Well-nourished individuals have ingested 1000 mg (1 gm) or more of pure amygdalin every day without any evidence of "side effects". In one case study an 11-month-old girl was reported accidentally to have ingested up to 5 amygdalin tablets (500 mg). The child became listless within a half hour of ingestion and vomited. Breathing became irregular and her state of consciousness became altered. An hour after ingestion she was in shock and died approximately 72 h following ingestion in spite of hospital treatment. Some sources claim that the death was the result of treatment. In another case-study a 17-year-old girl suffering from cancer made a practice of taking, instead of radiotherapy, four ampules of laetrile (3 g amygdalin) intravenously. One day she swallowed about 1 gm of laetrile. Shortly after ingestion, a severe headache and dizziness developed, and she collapsed. Her breathing became labored, her pupils dilated, and coma followed. All symptoms occurred within 10 minutes after ingestion. She died 24 h after ingestion. In Anatolia (Turkey) there were 9 cases of cyanide intoxication of children due to the ingestion of wild apricot seeds (217 mg HCN/100g) were reported. The victims had probably eaten more than 10 seeds. Also, others reported poisoning in studies after consuming a relative large amount of peach seeds or bitter almonds. Quantitative figures on cyanogenic glycoside or cyanide intake are not omitted. Important: See Laetrile, cyanogenic glycosides, Apple seeds

Amylase enzymes

An enzyme that helps digest carbohydrates (starch and glycogen) into simple sugar glucose and maltose for energy. Amylase is made in the the salivary glands and in the pancreas.

Anthocyanidins

are water soluble flavinoid pigments that are found in many plants and are responsible for the autumn coloration of many leaves. They are also powerful antioxidants. Cyanidin and malvidin both inhibit COX-1 and COX-2 enzymes. Malvidin and pelargonidin both exhibited inhibitory action against the proliferation of some human tumor cell lines.

Apple seeds

contain vitamin B17 (Laetrile) is a nitriloside, which occurs naturally in fruit seeds, some berries, as well as flax seed. It was presented as a cure for cancer several decades ago by Dr. Ernst T. Krebs. Other seeds containing nitrilosides are bitter almond, apricot, blackthorn, cherry, nectarine, peach and plum. See Laetrile, cyanogenic glycosides, Details under Amygdalin

Antineoplastons

Refers to mixtures of peptides, amino acids, and other organic substances that were first isolated from human urine and blood by Stanislaw Burzynski. Claims of antineoplastons to treat a variety of cancers are based on the belief that they promote the body's natural defenses against cancer. This modality has finally over come extensive suppression.

Arachidonic acid

is an omega-6 fatty acid that is present in corn oil as well as other vegetable oils and has been shown to **promote cancer development** while omega-3 fatty acids are known to inhibit cancer formation and growth. This is a solid indication that corn oil and possibly some other vegetable oils should be avoided. See Omega-6 fatty acids.

Artemisinin

is also known as wormwood, which has been used to fight malaria and other parasites. It has the characteristic of reacting with iron, which accumulates in certain parasites and some cancers as well.

Asparagus

was a popular remedy for kidney stones back in the 1800's. It was later found to have an influence on cancer and its popularity is increasing. One recipe suggest using canned or cooked asparagus to make a puree which is refrigerated. Daily consumption of 4 tablespoonfuls the puree is believed to be sufficient. Interestingly, asparagus contains significant amounts of histones which are important in binding specific genes for the regulation of cellular activity.

Aspirin

taken 2 times daily (325 mg) has been shown to reduce the risk of certain cancers by as much as 40 percent. Ibuprofen is less effective and acetaminophen (Tylenol) shows almost no effectiveness. Aspirin is an NSAID and is effective in reducing inflammation and increases blood flow. It is also an inhibitor of COX-1and COX-2 enzymes. Since aspirin has been shown to reduce the risk of cardiovascular illness, daily use should be strongly considered.

is a carotenoid and is the pigment that gives salmon its pink color and also is the red pigment found in crustaceans such as shrimp, lobsters, and crabs. It is also the chemical that gives flamingos their pink feathers. It is considered chemically to be a better anti-oxidant than beta-carotene which it is similar to. It is reported to be 10 times as effective as an anti-oxidant than other carotenoids and 100 times as effective as vitamin E. It also may be extremely important as it can cross the blood-brain barrier, which many other anti-oxidants are not able to do. It is also considered to be non-toxic. Significant amounts are available in Norwegian krill oils Such as Neptune Krill Oil.

Astragalus

has been used as an **immune booster** in Chinese medicine for thousands of years. It is also a blood thinner so caution should be used when taking this herb. It has been shown in one small study to boost the immune system in cancer patients. Other studies show that it not only boosts the production of white blood cells but also increases the activity of T-lymphocytes. It also appears to increase the production of interferon. Astragaloside IV (AGS-IV) is isolated from the roots of astragalus and are extraordinarily effective anti-neoplastic substance that is currently being studied for pancreatic cancer with good results.

Berberine

is a plant alkaloid that has been found to be a strong COX-2 inhibitor and is found in various herbs including Goldenseal and Barberry. It is antibacterial and anti-fungal and appears to reduce the adhesion of microbes to body tissues as well. It is helpful in reducing Candida infections as well as being effective against other parasites. It also lowers cholesterol and triglycerides. About 3 – 250-mg capsules daily may be beneficial. Check bottle label for best dosage.

Beta-Glucan

beta-1,3-D-glucan has been found to **stimulate the immune system**, especially macrophage activity, natural killer cells, and T-lymphocytes. It also shows significant anti-tumor activity including increased tumor necrosis factor. According to some sources, it is important that the B-glucan you buy is immuno assayed for effectiveness. It is the quality rather than quantity that is important with this supplement. Some users will take is 2 to 3 grams daily taken 20 minutes before food. As there are variations between brands, check bottle label for best dosage.

beta-sitosterol

An anti-tumor sterol, lends credence to its traditional use to treat abscesses and tumors of the abdomen, eyes, and liver. It is also highly rated for reducing prostate inflammation and prostate cancer.

Bicarbonate of soda

is currently being promoted by Dr. Simoncini of Italy to eliminate cancer. He feels that cancer is basically a fungal infection and that Sodium Bicarbonate is very effective in eliminate it. At the very least, the **bicarbonate of soda is contributing to the alkalinity** of the body, helping to eliminate cancer that way. It is also used frequently to help the kidneys recover from damage as a result of excessively high levels of acid in the blood. The 2009 Journal of the American Society of *Astragalus* 60Nephrology revealed a study of 134 patients with advanced kidney disease. Taking baking soda daily dramatically slowed down the progression of kidney disease, resulting, in some cases, no need for dialysis.

Bindweed

is a common garden weed that appears to fight cancer by **inhibiting angiogenesis**. Angiogenesis is the process of developing new blood vessels which are necessary for continued cancer growth. It appears that bindweed is almost 100 times as effective as shark cartilage in its inhibition of angiogenesis.

Black cumin seeds

are known from ancient times, mentioned in the Old Testament and found in the tomb of Tutankhamen. The seeds are used in cooking and are revered for their healing powers. They are rich in fatty acids such as oleic acid, linoleic acid, and lenolenic acid. Black cumin has no significant side effects when taken in normal dosage, even with long term usage. Black cumin is valuable and effective as an anti-parasitic. It is sometimes taken with garlic as a harmonizer and may also be taken with royal jelly. Thymoquinone, an extract of Black Cumin has been tested and found to be effective in stopping the growth of pancreatic cancer as well as causing apoptosis.

is a corrosive salve, often referred to as "escharotics" because they produce a thick, dry scab called an "eschar" on the skin. These salves have been in use to treat cancer dating back hundreds of years, perhaps even to ancient times and were commonly used during the 18th and 19th centuries. The idea of these products is to apply them to cancers that are close to the surface of the skin where the salve can directly attack and kill them. There are many positive testimonials as well as some reported serious injuries from the use of black salve. Use sensibility, do not apply to large areas if you use this and apply only small amounts to localized lesions. The main constituents of black salve are blood root and zinc chloride. Some recipes include chaparral or pine tar. As can be seen, this product can be quite corrosive.

Blood Root

(*Sanguinaria canadensis*) is an herb that grows wild in eastern North America and has long been use by the North American Indian tribes. It is named for the reddish-orange roots that it stores its toxic sap in. The Indians use the juice of the root as face paint, so in its basic, unconcentrated form, it must not have had many bad effects. More recently, it has been used as a folk medicine for the removal of warts and skin tags. It is also effective in low concentrations against skin fungus, ringworm, etc. It has definite anti-microbial properties but should be considered toxic even though it has been used as an emetic. <u>Sanguinarine</u> is the main toxin and kills animal cells by blocking the action of Na^+/K^+-ATPase so that it will kill skin on contact. It is not specific for cancer as claimed by some and may cause sever pain as well as deep lesions that take months to heal. Small amounts applied to localized skin cancers such as melanoma may have some benefits but extreme caution is advised.

Bromelain

is a collection of proteolytic enzymes and several other substances such as peroxidase, acid phosphatase, and protease inhibitors that is normally extracted from the pineapple plant. It is effective as a digestive aid when taken with meals and is anti-inflammatory. It also contains at least 2 substances that have been shown to be anti-cancer agents. Bromelain can help to remove dead tissue and has also been shown to improve immune function and aid in wound healing. It is not recommended to take bromelain if you have ulcers and there are some reported allergies to it. Otherwise, it is recommended by some sources to take 500 mg 3 times daily as a pain moderator. The effectiveness as a pain moderator is reduced when bromelain is taken with meals.

Burdock Root

was known to the ancient Greeks and has been used as a remedy all over the world, and is a main constituent of **Essiac Tea** and of the **Hoxsey** formula. It is known to lower blood sugar but its main use is as an alkalizer. It is also reported to exhibit diuretic effects as well as having anti-fungal and antimicrobial properties. Also it is a key herb in Blessed Hildegard of Bingen's 12th century internal tonic for cancer. Burdock is sometimes combined with yellow dock and sarsaparilla. Experimental extracts have shown the following effects: antibacterial, antifungal, antifurunculous, anti-tumor, diuretic, estrogenic, hypoglycemic. Burdock is also said to contain antiviral compounds specific to fighting AIDS, but verification currently lacking.

Calcium

is an alkaline mineral that is extremely important to good health and to fighting cancer. In areas with high calcium content in the water, there is often a significantly lower rate of certain cancers and a longer life span. It has been shown to reduce blood pressure and to reduce colon tumors. Dosage may be 1200 to 1500 mg daily for best results but this should be reduced when high calcium foods are eaten. Calcium should be balanced with magnesium and vitamin D3 supplementation is beneficial as is vitamin K2. Exceeding 2000 mg daily appears to increase the risk of prostate cancer. See vitamin D

Cancell

also known as Cantron and Protocell was developed in the early 1930's as an anti-cancer therapy under the name Entelev. It was re-introduced in the 1980's as Cancell and was quickly labeled as ineffective by the NCI but has since been shown to have strong anti-oxidant activity. The stated purpose of Cancell is to starve cancer cells of energy, thereby causing them to die a slow death. Due to FDA action Cancell may not be produced, sold, or given away in the United States. It is available in Europe and many other areas around the world. Some studies have shown Cancell to be **twice as effective as Taxol** (a standard chemotherapy drug) with far less negative aspects. Cantron and Protocell are available as supplements.

is a carotenoid substance with anti-oxidant properties. When used as a tanning agent, it has been reported to cause retinopathy due to deposits of yellow pigmentation in the retina. It is considered reversible once the supplement is no longer ingested. There have also been reports of liver damage.

Capsaicin

is the active compound in many peppers that give it its heat. Capsaicin is strongest in habanero peppers. As a note of warning, habanero peppers are extremely hot! It has been found that capsaicin can induce apoptosis in certain lines of cancer cells including some prostate and pancreatic cancers. It also halts or reduces growth of other cells lines such as certain prostate cancers. It has been shown to increase the presence of stomach and intestinal cancers in laboratory tests. A capsaicin infusion can be made by placing 1 tsp. of cayenne pepper into 1 cup of boiling water. This is then diluted 1 tsp. to a glass of water and this is consumed 3 to 4 times daily. Others actually swallow a whole habanero pepper daily or drink habanero juice. It would be necessary to eat a habanero daily in order to have full effect for a 200 pound man. This has been shown to reduce prostate cancer cells in mice by 80 percent. It also appears to work with lung cancers as well as with pancreatic cancer. Following is a recipe. Place 1 grated habanero on bread, then place 2 grated cloves of fresh garlic on bread. Cover both generously with real cow butter and eat. Some sources recommend 1 to 2 tbsp of cod liver oil daily or evening primrose oil depending on the persons condition. If you can not tolerate peppers, try substituting fresh ginger in place of the peppers. Either the peppers, garlic, or the ginger must be grated freshly each day. Use only real cow butter as it contains specific oils that are needed. As a final note, people who live in areas where large amounts of spicy foods are eaten have lower rates of cancer.

Carotenoids

are the pigments that give many fruits and vegetables their bright red, orange, yellow, and green colors and provide a wide range of antioxidant and cancer inhibiting properties. Do not rely on just B-carotene. Lycopene, lutein, zeaxanthin, canthaxanthin, beta-cryptoxanthin, fucoxanthin, astaxanthin, capsanthin, crocetin, phytoene, and alpha-carotene all produce beneficial results and many are converted to vitamin A in the body. Suggested daily amounts from various sources are 10-30 mg of lycopene, 15 to 40 mg of leutine, 10 to 20 mg of sulphoraphane, 25000 IU of alpha and beta-carotene combined daily for short periods of time. Leutine intake has been associated with reduced colon cancer. Try to get all of these amounts from food if at all possible because when taken in supplement form, they are not as effective. Additionally, when consumed in foods, there are other beneficial substances included that may be missing from the supplements. It is recommended to avoid the baby carrots because they are often made from larger carrots and then soaked in chlorine solution to kill germs. This chlorine is very damaging to immunity. Also, one study in China suggests that drinking alcohol with high levels of carotinoids may increase lung cancer risk. In another study, high serum β-carotene concentrations were associated with increased risk for aggressive, clinically relevant prostate cancer.

Castor oil

is composed mostly of ricinoleic acid, which is a fatty acid, thought to be responsible for castor oil's healing properties. It was used for medical reasons in Ancient Egypt, Greece, Rome, Persia, and China. In modern times, Castor oil has even been used to treat multiple sclerosis, arthritis, epilepsy, appendicitis, colitis, and Parkinson's Disease among many other illnesses. It is considered to boost immunity and boost function of the Thymus gland.

Cats claw

contains several alkaloid compounds that have been shown to stimulate immune response. Two small cancer studies have also demonstrated that cats claw extract may reduce some tumors.

Cayenne

is a form of pepper and contains capsaicin, carotenoids, flavinoids, as well as several vitamins. It has been used for pain relief. Capsaicin has been shown to induce apoptosis in certain cancers.

Cesium Chloride

is popular and effective among very late stage cancer sufferers (less than 1 to 2 months' survival expected) but there are serious risks associated with using this. This is possibly the most effective late stage anti-cancer alternative therapy presently available although it is rejected by the cancer industry. Cesium is very specifically and rapidly absorbed into cancer cells causing rapid death of the cancer cells. The problem is that the death of a large number of cells at once can overload the liver, kidneys, spleen, and other organs. The effects of die-off in this case can be severe and may result in organ failure, leading to death. Cesium salts may also cause heart irregularities. For this reason, it should be administered gradually and potassium should be taken with it. In cases of early stage cancer, it may be very effective but at this time has not been tried. It is certainly recommended that anyone who uses Cesium or Rubidium salts to treat cancer should have good liver function and very good kidney function. To help remove toxins from the body, colonics and coffee enemas are suggested. In extreme cases, dialysis may also be suggested. Reportedly, in areas with high Cesium or Rubidium intake, cancer is very rare.

Chaga Mushroom

Has been used as a folk medicine for cancer and other ailments. The chaga mushroom grows on birch trees. In addition to interfering with the metastasis of cancer, it is also believed to contain a number of immune boosting substances as the mature mushroom contains over 200 phytonutrients.

Chaparral Tea

contains a potent antioxidant nordihydroguaiaretic acid (NDGA) and is an old Indian remedy for cancer. It is made from the twigs and leaves of the creosote brush. One substance, tetramethyl-O-nordihydroguaiaretic acid (M4N) that is found in chaparral tea has been shown to reduce tumors of head and neck cancer, which are difficult to remove. In all cases of the study, the tumors were successfully shrunk but there was extreme pain and other side effects from the injections. While there have been some positive reports from the use of this tea against cancer, caution should be used as it has also been implicated in liver problems.

Chlorella

has not been shown to directly stop or kill cancer cells so the assumption is that it works by boosting the immune system. In this respect, chlorella is very important nutritionally as it contains large amounts of necessary vitamins, amino acids, minerals, and other important nutrients. It has been shown to boost survival rates significantly in various studies. Taking a fresh source of chlorella is highly recommended.

Chlorophyll

has been shown to bind many carcinogens so that they are not absorbed into the body. It is also occasionally absorbed where it can have additional anti cancer effects. It is also believed to be a powerful detoxifier.

Chymotrypsin

is a proteolytic enzyme produced along with trypsin by the pancreas. Both are valuable in removing the proteins that surround tumors and a deficiency of these is common in many cancer cases. These proteins are extensively used in the digestion of meats and this is likely one of the main reasons that a diet of all fruits and vegetables is successful in beating cancer. Any meat ingested will remove these enzymes from the body and reduce the amount available for cancer fighting. There is an advantage to taking these in supplement form for many cancer types, especially pancreatic and liver cancers. Bromelain and papain are two additional proteolytic enzymes that may be of benefit.

Cilantro

is a popular component of Mexican, Latin, Caribbean, and eastern meals that contains limonene, borneol, as well as caffeic acid, and chlorogenic acid, both of which are antioxidants. Cilantro has been shown in studies to reduce some skin cancers and is anti-inflammatory and antibiotic. One proposed idea is that Cilantro removes cancer causing heavy metals such as Mercury from the body. Intake of just one spoonful of cilantro daily is suggested to reduce the danger of skin cancer by about 30%.

Cinnamon

is a known glucose-insulin modifier that improves insulin sensitivity, and it has long been used by diabetics to fight insulin resistance. There are compounds in cinnamon that appear to emulate insulin and therefore can be a limited replacement for insulin. Cinnamon has also been shown to stop cell proliferation in both leukemia and lymphoma through in-vitro studies. In addition to lowering glucose, cinnamon has also been shown in studies to lower cholesterol and triglycerides. Beneficial amounts of cinnamon range from a quarter teaspoon a day to one teaspoonful three times daily. It is best taken in capsule form with water about twenty to thirty minutes before a meal. Cinnamon contains water-soluble compounds are called procyanidins (type A), and MHCP (methylhydroxychalcone polymer), both of which are polyphenols. Cinnamon with honey can have additional benefits as research in Japan and in Australia has shown that this combination has successfully cured bone cancer and stomach cancer. Certain cinnamon products are high in coumarin content that can cause liver damage and can also interact with drugs .

Cloves

have been shown to help regulate glucose and to reduce cholesterol and triglycerides. Researchers at the UAE University studied clove extract on four cancer cell lines, **T-cell lymphoma**, **cervical carcinoma**, **human neuroblastoma** and **human leukemia** and found the clove extracts do have effectiveness in these cases. In India, scientists found that cloves inhibited lung cancers in mouse lungs. The study showed that cloves increased p53 and Bax, reduced Bcl-2, and inhibits the COX-2 enzyme along with , cMyc and Hras. Cloves contain eugenol, caryophyllene, and tannins

Cod Liver Oil

Is an excellent source of the omega 3 fatty acids, eicosapentaenoic acid (EPA) and docosahexaenoic acid (DHA). Since it contains natural sources of Vitamin A and D, it helps reduce your risk for cancer.

also known as ubiquinone and also as ubiquinol, inhibits cancer proliferation and progression as well as reduces infection, liver and cardiac damage. It also helps boost the immune system and is important as a free radical scavenger. Low levels of CoQ10 in the blood have been directly associated with cardiac failure, cancer, and with liver disease. CoQ10 is normally produced in the body, especially in the liver. The production of CoQ10 is a multi-step process that requires at least 7 different vitamins and several trace elements. If any of these is deficient, production of CoQ10 is reduced. Production is also seriously reduced in cases of liver ailment and when certain statin drugs are used. It should be noted that CoQ10 is extremely important in mitochondrial function and its absence will severely impair cellular respiration. Also, one of the observed characteristics of cancerous cells it that this mitochondrial function is suppressed. CoQ10 may help restore some of that function thereby reducing the spread of cancer. CoQ10 is also especially important to those who are using statin drugs to lower cholesterol. CoQ10 should not be used with some of the other therapies and in some cases may accelerate some cancer growth. Daily consumption of 200 to 400 mg is suggested when CoQ10 is used. Ubiquinol is a form that is more easily absorbed giving about eight times higher blood levels so that as little as 50 mg of this form is needed. Some individuals have taken larger dosages but care should be used and larger dosages should be taken under the direction of a medical professional who is knowledgeable in respect to CoQ10. Co-

Q10 should not be used in conjunction with graviola, paw-paw, or other ATP inhibitors.

Coffee enemas

are used to help eliminate toxins from the body and to stimulate the liver. They are used as an integral part of several alternative therapies. Organically grown coffee is brewed as for drinking, brought to body temperature, placed into a enema bag, and introduced into the colon and intestines where it should be held for 20 to 30 minutes. Coffee enemas are used by many for general health and users often report all over general improvement in feeling and health. The caffeine stimulates the intestines while other components help draw toxins from the body as help remove old fecal material from the lining of the intestines and colon. Why organically grown? Coffee is grown in foreign countries where pesticides are largely unregulated.

Colonics

is the process of flushing out the colon, similar to enemas. Cleansing the colon can aid health in general as well as immunity. It also aids in the removal of toxins from the body.

Conjugated Linoleic Acid (CLA)

is actually a family of many forms of linoleic acid that inhibits tumor formation and metastasis and also encourages apoptosis. The natural form of CLA comes from the meat and dairy products of grass fed animals and it is an important fatty acid. It helps in reducing the amount of fat in the body while increasing muscle, lowers cholesterol and triglycerides, and lowers insulin resistance. When taking the synthetic form which is inferior, recommended intake is 1 to 6 – 1000 mg capsules daily. The synthetic supplements have higher levels of the trans-10, cis-12 isomer that have been linked to health problems. It is interesting that CLA is a trans-fat that has actual health benefits.

Cottage cheese and flaxseed oil

is the basic formula for the **Budwig cancer protocol**. Reportedly, this protocol has a high rate of remission with some cancers. Dr. Johanna Budwig, PhD., first proposed this protocol in 1951 as she had found that the blood of many cancer patients was low in certain fats and essential fatty acids. This diet combines alpha linolenic acid (precursor for omega-3 fatty acids) with protein from the cottage cheese to make the oils water-soluble. One cup of organic cottage cheese is blended with 1-1/2 ounce to 5 ounces of flaxseed oil and natural flavorings such as figs, pears, dates, apples, or grapes. Cayenne, garlic, or red pepper may be added as may ground flaxseed. Also, unrefined cold pressed walnut, linseed, sunflower, and poppy seed oils may be substituted.

Cryptoxanthin

is a carotenoid and an active antioxidant. Tests in China show that higher serum levels of B-cryptoxanthin correlate with reduced lung cancer in smokers. Some of these studies indicate that B-cryptoxanthin is more critical in reducing the occurrence of cancer than is vitamin-C or B-carotene. Because B-cryptoxanthin occurs naturally along side of B-carotene this may be one reason that tests using purified B-carotene have not produced the expected results.

directly inhibits the COX-2 enzyme and can can interfere with the activity of the transcription factor <u>NF-κB</u>. It also inhibits TXA2 and as a result reduces tumor blood supply and lessens metastasis. It also inhibits 5-lipoxygenase. Another study indicates that curcumin may inhibit <u>mTOR</u> complex I. It is known to be anti-carcinogenic, anti-inflammatory, and a free radical scavenger. It also has a low toxicity and few side effects. According to some sources, suggested dosage for cancer is up to 4 - 900 mg capsules 3 x daily. A small amount of piperine or Bioperine should be included to help increase absorption. A new improved formula, Super Bio-Curcumin is available that has 7 times the absorption levels. Several studies have been completed completed showing the safety and tolerability of curcumin in colorectal cancer patients.

cyanogenic glycosides

are compounds often found in many plants that have a C=N bound to a glycoside (basically a sugar based molecule). A common example is Vitamin B17, also referred to as Laetrile and Amygdalin. The concern is that the Cyanide radical can be released into the body causing cyanide poisoning. This can be a problem in ruminants because their second stomach contains bacteria that can break down the cyanide bond and the pH is often more alkaline than the stomach of other animals. Much of the toxicity concern is raised by the fact that cattle and other ruminants die from cyanide poisoning from the breakdown of cyanogenic glycosides more frequently. I have spent extensive time researching possible deaths to humans from cyanogenic glycosides but have only found a few actual cases that have been reasonably documented. See **Amygdalin**. Among the substances that are warned against ingesting are apple seeds, peach seeds, apricot seeds, avocado pits, and even flax seed. Sources claim that 2 or 3 apples seeds would be deadly, but there are many people who eat a teaspoon or even a tablespoonful daily without illness. The truth is that if these seeds were so deadly, there would be a lot of dead horses because horses love apples and eat the entire fruit. Cows and sheep will get sick and die from this because they are ruminates. The problem with these warnings is that the human digestive system is too acid to allow the free production of cyanide except from metal-cyanides such as potassium cyanide. Normal cells in the human body do not convert the cyanogenic glycosides into cyanide but the interesting thing is that tumor cells do so that they are specifically killed by the reaction of cyanogenic glycosides with the enzyme beta-glucosidase which releases the cyanide inside of the cancer cells. Many plants bear beta-glucosidase in their cells, which is released by chewing, but the acidity of the stomach will quickly neutralize the beta-glucosidase. One problem is that bacteria in the intestines can convert cyanogenic glycosides to cyanide if the intestines are allowed to become alkaline enough. The warning here is that you should not ingest any alkaline substance such as cesium chloride, sodium bicarbonate, calcium carbonate, or any other antacid when consuming plants with cyanogenic glycosides and always use caution. It is probably best to take these cyanogenic compounds without food because the more food, the more acid that it neutralizes. Start out with small amounts if you go this route. Taking the methylcobalamin form of vitamin B12 can help neutralize excess HCN that is produced in the cells. MSM (methyl-sulfonyl methionine) is also reported to help neutralize any adverse effects. Also, cyanide causes an increase in blood glucose and lactic acid levels and a decrease in the ATP/ADP ratio. This indicates a shift from aerobic to anaerobic metabolism. Cyanide apparently activates glycogenolysis and shunts glucose to the pentose phosphate pathway resulting in a decrease in the rate of glycolysis and inhibiting the tricarboxylic acid cycle. One last note again, use caution. See Apple seeds, Amygdalin, Laetrile

Dandelion

root powder has been reported to eliminate cancer in some cases. A couple of recipes suggested that, one should dig up the entire plant and remove the leaves at the crown. Do not wash but shake as much dirt off as is possible. Dry the roots for several days at about 100 degrees F. Do not overheat. Once the roots are completely dry, grind them up with a mortar and pestle being careful not to loose the dust or fine powder. Mix ½ tsp. with water only and drink all of it once a day. It does take time for results, as it appears to work as an immunity builder. Dandelion has been used in many traditional medical systems, including Native American and traditional Arabic medicine and has been most commonly used to treat liver diseases, kidney diseases, and spleen problems. In 2008, a study on breast and prostate cancer cells, researchers found that dandelion leaf extract slowed the growth of breast cancer cells and stopped the spread of prostate cancer cells. Neither dandelion flower extract nor dandelion root extract had any effect on either type of cancer cell. Researchers found that dandelion extracts significantly reduced the blood sugar level in diabetic rats and might be a useful tool against that disease. Since cancer is so hungry for blood sugar, this might be part of its effectiveness. Scientists were able to prevent skin cancer in mice, using dandelion extract suggesting that dandelion "could be a valuable chemotherapy preventive agent". It has been demonstrated by Chinese researchers that dandelion can restore the three major types of immune functions: cell-mediated, humoral, and non-specific immunity. Dandelion also inhibits TNF-alpha, a harmful natural substance, that is involved in cachexia, the wasting syndrome of cancer. It has anti-inflammatory effects, particularly noticeable in the central nervous system. Some of the notable components of dandelion extracts are Caffeic acid, linoleic, linolenic, oleic and palmitric acids, coumarins , Luteolin-7-glucoside and luteolin-7-diglucoside, Carotenoids, choline, inulin, pectin, phytosterols, and triterpenes.

DHA

docosahexaenoic acid is an omega-3 fatty acid that is important in overall nutrition and has been shown to have definite anti-cancer properties. It has been shown to inhibit cancer cell growth and cause cancer cell apoptosis in some cell lines as well as improving the effectiveness of chemotherapy drugs such as cisplatin. It is also important for reduction of arteriosclerosis and for proper neural function. In studies, it has been shown to reduce or even stop the toxic kidney side-effects of cancer therapy. It can reduce CRP (C-reactive protein) and serves as a rejuvinator for antioxidants. Fish oil with high EPA/DHA content can reduce the risk of colon cancer and other cancers by inhibiting the COX-2 enzyme. A study in 2000 showed that DHA inhibited the growth of Melanoma cells by 50 percent in vitro. Another study found that high EPA/DHA supplementation increased the life expectancy of pancreatic cancer by almost 2 times and actually contributed to weight gain. Another study also showed either weight gain or reduced weight loss in stage 4 cancer patients who took up to 12 gm of fish oil daily. It is advised in several studies to take vitamin E along with the EPA/DHA supplements while other studies claim that vitamin E reduces the level of apoptosis generated by DHA. DHA should be as fresh as possible as oxidation reduces its effectiveness. Taking vitamin D is also beneficial. See: Fish Oil, Omega-3 Fatty acids, EPA, Vitamin D, Vitamin E, Omega 6 fatty acids, alpha lipoic acid.*Dihydroepiandosterone (*

DHEA)

is an anti-aging pro-hormone that has significant value in the management of cancer including, reduction of fatigue, boosting of immune function, improvement of brain function and protection of brain cells, reduction of cachexia, and reduction of inflammation. As it is a precursor for many hormones used by the human body and some used by certain cancers, there may be negative effects in those cases where the cancers are hormone sensitive. It should possibly be avoided in ovarian, breast, prostate, and other hormone influenced cancers.

Digestive enzyme

supplements may be beneficial in reducing fatigue in cancer patients. Certain digestive enzyme have been shown to break down the coating that some cancer cells use to protect themselves. At the very least, digestive enzymes are important in improving the digestive processes and the absorption of nutrients. They may also have additional benefits. Pancreatic enzymes and hormones have been reputed to be effective against pancreatic cancer in some cases as well as against some other cancers..

Dimethyl Sulfoxide (DMSO)

is an anti-inflammatory and an excellent transporter of therapies into cancer cells as it is considered to be a universal solvent. While many US doctors frown on using DMSO, it is used extensively overseas without any significant reported problems. It has been found to increase the effectiveness of certain therapies. Some reports are found on the Internet where DMSO is mixed with Curcumin for effectiveness in certain brain cancers.

Ellagic acid

is a polyphenolic anti-oxidant that is found in many fruits and vegetables. Grapes, red raspberries, pomegranate, strawberries, and blueberries are major sources. It has been shown to slow the growth of cancers in the laboratory and may cause apoptosis in some cancers. A cup of red raspberries once or twice daily should provide sufficient serum levels of ellagic acid. More than twice that amount of strawberries or walnuts would be required. Researchers found that rats that consumed 5% to 10% of their diet as freeze-dried black raspberries and strawberries showed dramatic reductions in the growth of precancerous cells and tumor progression . In another study, the berries reduced colon cancer growth by 80%. Yet another study demonstrated that Ellagic acid is causing G-arrest within 48 hours (inhibiting and stopping mitosis-cancer cell division), and apoptosis (normal cell death) within 72 hours, for breast, pancreas, esophageal, skin, colon and prostate cancer cells.

English Ivy

leaf extract may have anti-mutagenic (anticancer) and antioxidant properties., based on preliminary animal studies. Falcarinol, which is a fatty alcohol found in carrots, red ginseng (*Panax ginseng*) and ivy, that protects roots from fungal diseases, and other polyacetylenes. In studies, Falcarinol proved to be the most active compound with a pronounced toxicity against acute lymphoblastic leukemia cell line CEM-C7H2. The leaves and fruits also contain the saponic glycoside hederagenin which, if ingested, can cause breathing difficulties and coma.

is another plant in which the seeds, twigs and wilted leaves of the plant contain the cyanogenic glycoside, amygdalin.

Entelev

is the original name for the products today known as Cancell, Cantron, and Protocell. See: Cancell.

Enzyme

therapies utilize various natural enzymes to help defeat cancer. Some of the enzymes used are bromelain, pancreatic enzymes (trypsin and chymotrypsin), papain, and other digestive enzymes. The theory is that the enzymes help breakdown certain proteins that protect the cancer cells from the immune system. It is suspected by some that eating meat reduces the amount of enzymes available in the body for fighting cancers. Additionally, taking digestive enzymes improves the digestion process.

EPA

eicosapentaenoic acid is an omega-3 fatty acid that is important in overall nutrition and produces cancer cell apoptosis in vivo in certain cancers such as pancreatic. It is considered as an essential fatty acid because while it can be produced in small amounts in the body, the process is long and difficult. It is important in keeping the heart and arteries in good condition. A good source is from Salmon and some other fish. EPA should be as fresh as possible as oxidation reduces its effectiveness. See DHA, Fish oil, Omega-3 fatty acid, arachadonic acid, alpha lipoic acid.

is a brewers yeast extract noted for its immunity boosting abilities. Tests show that EpiCor boosts the activity of NK cells.

Essential Fatty Acids (EFAs)

inhibit COX-2 enzyme, reduce or prevent cachexia, improve the effectiveness of other therapies, and regulate cell division. The presence of fatty acids is critically important in the maintenance of cardiac function. Especially important are the omega-3 fatty acids, EPA or eicosapentaenoic acid and DHA or docosahexaenoic acid which are mainly derived from animal sources and fish oils. These fatty acids can not be synthesized in the human body as they are produced from Alpha-Linolenic acid and Linoleic acid, neither of which can be synthesized in the human body without the addition of these precursors. Most important sources are fish oil and flax seed oil. Suggested dosage varies from 6 – 1000 mg capsules a day to 8 or more 1000-mg capsules daily depending on the type and source. See cottage cheese and flaxseed oil.

Essiac Tea

is from an old American Indian recipe and was discovered by Renee Caisse. It is a tea made from four to eight natural growing herbs that have been shown to have several beneficial properties. Formulas vary between producers, but any of these should be beneficial. The taste is bitter but essiac is a strong alkalizer. The drink I taken as an alkalizer and to cleanse the internal organs. It also contains numerous other valuable substances for boosting immunity. While it is an important part of any cancer therapy that may use it, it is probably not a cancer cure on its own. The main components are Sheep sorrel *(Rumex acetosella),* Slippery elm *(Ulmus fulva),* Burdock *(Arctium lappa), and* Rhubarb *(Rheum palmatum).*this is a cure that was introduced by a nurse, Rene Caisse, who learned about the herbal treatment from a prospector's wife who had survived breast cancer. The recipe originally came from Ojibway Indians, Native Americans of the area and was based on 4 main herbs. These herbs were burdock root, sheep sorrel, slippery elm bark, and Indian rhubarb root (some sources say Turkish Rhubarb root), all of which grow wild in North America. Other recipes add ingredients such as kelp.

When she found out about the healing properties of these herbs, Caisse started treating people, using the recipe, for free. She never charged for her work. Once word spread, she was allowed to set up a clinic in Ontario and with the assistance of doctors, continued to treat patients, producing many testimonials. She did not have any clinical trials and there has not been any serious clinical trials to date. The reason for this is that Essiac Tea, no matter how powerful or effective, is not profitable to the cancer industry. In laboratory tests, Sheep Sorrel and Burdock Root have been shown to kill cancer cells.

While I am not fighting cancer, I have used Essiac as a herbal immune supporter, on and off, for many years. I would consider Essiac Tea as a good choice for stage 1,2, or 3 cancers but it is not likely strong enough for a stage 4 treatment on its own. I certainly would not hesitate adding it to whatever stage 4 protocol that I was following. I certainly think that it would be beneficial to those who are recovering from chemotherapy or radiation treatments. Essiac Tea works slowly to help remove some of the actual causes of cancer so do not expect an overnight miracle or dramatic tumor shrinkage in short time.

Even if it does not cure cancer, Essiac Tea is beneficial because it contains many nutrients and helps to support your immune system without major side effects. So just buy Essiac Tea for its health benefits and for your happiness.

The place where I buy my Essiac Tea has been suppressed by the FTC and no longer sells Essiac as a cure but if you call them, you can get it as a herbal supplement.

For other information please visit http://www.cancertutor.com/Cancer/ Essiac.html . They have the most thorough website on fighting cancer, however, there are complaints that some of the clinics that they promote are financial influences.

This formula is a transcription of Mary McPherson's affidavit:

6 ½ cups of burdock root (cut)*

1 pound of sheep sorrel herb powdered

1/4 pound of slippery elm bark powdered

1 ounce of Turkish rhubarb root powdered

Mix these ingredients thoroughly and store in glass jar in dark dry cupboard.

Take a measuring cup, use 1 ounce of herb mixture to 32 ounces of water depending on the amount you want to make.

I use 1 cup of mixture to 8 x 32 = 256 ounces of water. Boil hard for 10 minutes (covered) then turn off heat but leave sitting on warm plate over night (covered).

In the morning heat steaming hot and let settle a few minutes, then strain through fine strainer into hot sterilized bottles and sit to cool. Store in dark cool cupboard. Must be refrigerated when opened. When near the last when its thick pour in a large jar and sit in frig overnight then pour off all you [can] without sediment.

Estrogen

increases the risk of both breast cancer and uterine cancer. It is a well known activator of specific genes that code for the production of proteins that combine with lipids to bind cholesterol. Certain cells bear estrogen receptors that when estrogen binds to them, it will stimulate replication and proliferation. An example if the increase of endometrial cells in response to increased estrogen in preparation for pregnancy. Estrogen also stimulates the increase of mammary cells.

Fasting

is a part of some of the most effective alternative therapies and is often an accidental result of many chemo-therapies and radiation. Some of these alternative therapies call for fasting for 12 to 18 hours a day, drinking nothing but water during that period. In others, fruit and vegetable juices may be taken. The balance of the day, the diet consists of certain specified foods. I feel that it can be beneficial to fast even longer, one or two days to really clean the body out and starve the cancer cells. Do not over do it though and use care, especially if the cancer sufferer is emaciated or cachexic. After fasting, an Epsom salt flush will help remove additional toxins.

The Magic of the Epsom Salts Flush

There is a reason why Epsom salt is so good at cleaning out the intestines, because it actually causes a reverse flush by pulling water back through the intestinal walls. This in turn will break away bio-film and sludge that is not forced out by other laxatives.

Better than just flushing, before doing the Epsom salt flush, do a 24 hour water only fast. This weakens any microbes and parasites that may be in the intestines as well as putting extra water into the body so that there is plenty of water to help the reverse flush.

Additionally, at the end of the fast and at the beginning of the flush, I like to **zap using a zapper** that has at least 8 frequencies. It takes a full hour but it is better at destroying a wide range of microbes. I also prefer the 4 point contact, with 3 points positive. Only one or two frequencies is not going to be effective enough.

Finally, after flushing, taking a tablespoon of yogurt (at least 5 or 6 different strains of beneficial microbes), every 15 to 20 minutes for the next couple of hours will help to restore the intestinal flora.

A clean gut with beneficial microbes will do wonders for your health, longevity, and well being.

I generally start my water fast on Thursday night, zap and take Epsom salts on Friday night, followed with my yogurt, and stay home Saturday. You will want to stay very close to the commode.

For drinking, I generally mix 2 teaspoonful of good food grade Epsom Salt into a 8 to 12 ounce glass of water. I also add lemon for flavoring. Note that Epsom salt is very bitter. Some of the yuckiest stuff that I have ever taken. I also keep a separate glass of lemon water for that reason, to use as a chaser. It works very quickly and you will notice the difference. The result will be very yucky and smelly in most cases as it is cleaning out stuff that you would not believe. I generally do mine on Friday evening and stay home for the next 24 hours. Would hate for it to hit in public.

Before starting, take a picture of the Iris of your eyes. Then a couple of days after completing take another. Many people will see a significant difference. If you like the difference that you see, you can post before and after photos in the comments.

To me, the experience was almost like a right of passage and it can bring about change. At one point, I was a heavy soda drinker with a significant candida issue. After flushing I was immediately a water drinker, did not want sodas, It was definitely transformational although it was not the first time that I had taken Epsom salt. It was the first time that I had done the full protocol in sequence.

In Hulda Clark's protocol, she also adds Ozonated olive oil and grapefruit juice to help flush the gall bladder. This is also extremely beneficial

Feverfew

contains several COX-2 inhibitors and a lipoxygenase inhibitor. While it has been found to be effective against at least one form of leukemia, acute myelogenous leukemia (AML), it has traditionally been used for the reduction of fever, easing the pain of headaches and arthritis, and for treating digestive difficulties. It has also been used to treat menstrual irregularities and skin conditions. Feverfew is a platelet activity inhibitor so that care should be used if blood thinners are needed or if the person taking it has bleeding disorders. Do not take feverfew if you have a known allergy or hypersensitivity to chamomile, ragweed, yarrow, or other plants in the Asteraceae family. Follow dosage instructions on package..

Fish oil and fatty fish

consumption have been implicated in a **significant reduction in certain types of cancers** while lean white fish appears to have little or no effect. The main fatty fish are Salmon, Herring, Sardines, and Mackerel. Non-fatty fish include Tuna, Cod, Haddock, and fresh water fish. One study in Sweden compared the consumption of fatty fish with the occurrence of Kidney cancer. The group consuming fatty fish at least once a week experienced a 75 percent reduction in the occurrence of kidney cancer. In addition to the EPA and DHA that is present, vitamin D is also present in the fatty fish. Fish oil should be as fresh as possible as oxidation reduces its effectiveness. Many cancers are linked to vitamin D Deficiency. See DHA, EPA, Vitamin D, alpha lipoic acid, arachadonic acid, Omega-3 fatty acids.

Flaxseed oil

is high in alpha-linolenic acid, which is an omega-3 fatty acid. This is in turn a precursor for the manufacture of EPA and DHA in the human body. See Essential Fatty Acids. See: Budwig, cottage cheese and flax seed oil, DHA, EPA, Vitamin D, alpha lipoic acid, arachadonic acid, Omega-3 fatty acids.

Folic acid

helps to reduce anemia but also may increase cancer growth in some cases. There are many studies that indicate increased folic acid intake is extremely beneficial in slowing, reducing, or stopping cancer. It has been shown to help prevent certain cancers such as colon, breast, esophagus, and stomach cancer. It has been shown in one small study to reverse throat cancer. According to some sources, normal dosage is from 400 to 800 mcg daily. Some individuals take up to 3000 micrograms daily under a doctor's supervision. Folate should always be supplemented with vitamin B-12.

Fucoidan

is a sulfur containing polysaccharide that is found in many types of brown seaweed such as Kombu. It may also have some amounts of xylose, galactose, and glucuronic acid. Fucoidan has been shown in laboratory tests to cause apoptosis in tumor cells without affecting normal cells.

Garlic

the value of garlic has been touted for thousands of years. Scientific evidence shows that garlic stimulates lymphocyte production and effectiveness. It does thin the blood so this should be considered when garlic is used. Studies shows that the more fresh, raw garlic and / or onion that you eat the less chance that you have of developing many forms of cancer. The active ingredients appear to be several sulfur-containing compounds. Cooking can destroy some of these and some may be absent from powdered garlic. In a small pilot study, the test suggested that the more garlic people consumed, the lower the levels of the potential carcinogenic process were.

is a member of the cabbage family (brassicareae) that was imported from Europe as a medicinal herb more than a century ago and it has evolved into one of the better-known invasive species here in the U.S. It manufactures chemicals called glucosinolates, which makes it toxic to insects. The plant may decrease the germination of seeds from other plants, destroy organisms that certain varieties of trees need to live - and contaminate the ground where it grows. This is a strong indication that it has a lot of chemical activity.

Germanium

is a noted immune modulator and has been shown to increase immune response to cancer. It has also been shown to reduce pain in many cancer sufferers.

Ginger

is another herb that also contains multiple COX-2 inhibitors and lipoxygenase inhibitors and has been shown to kill ovarian cancer cells. It has more 5-lipoxygenase inhibitors than any other botanical reported to date. About 2 grams daily is recommended by some sources. Fresh ginger is often available in grocery stores. It is sometimes used to reduce nausea from chemotherapy or radiation therapy. One recent study showed a 45 percent reduction in severity of nausea in patients who took one quarter to one half teaspoon ginger before chemotherapy verses those who took a placebo. One component extracted from Ginger, [6]-gingerol, reduced the growth of human colorectal tumor cells in mice.

Glucophage

or metformin is an insulin sensitivity modulator. See: Metformin.

Glutamine

inhibits tumor growth, inhibits PGE2 synthesis, reduces infection, and increases NK cell activity. One noticeable condition of many cancer sufferers is low levels of glutamine. It is often taken in pill or capsule form with 500 to 1500 mg daily being considered safe. Healthcare professionals may prescribe 5000 to over 10000 mg daily.

Glutathione (GSH)

is an extremely powerful anti-oxidant and is functional in the rejuvenation of other anti-oxidants. It is so powerful in this respect that it is considered as an interference in the effectiveness of chemo-therapy. Also, in some other studies, high levels of glutathione in tumor cells has a negative effect on life expectancy of those tumor cells. Related enzymes are GSH-peroxidase, GSSG-reductase, and GSH-s-transferase P1-isoenzyme. GSSG-reductase is a replenishing enzyme while GSH-s-transferase P1-isoenzyme and GSH-peroxidase are depleting enzymes. One study on esophageal cancer showed that the replenishing enzymes were diminished. GSH-peroxidase will use GSH in the peroxidation of lipids. GST-P1 activity was enhanced but it was quickly transported out of the cancer cell into the blood. From this it is indicated that GSH is reduced in activity, at least in this cancer. The study used biopsies but did not indicate as to whether or not any chemotherapy had been administered which is important to any conclusions that may be drawn.

has been touted by some as the ultimate cure for cancer but there have not been any studies of significance to prove this. One study, in-vitro, a polysaccharide isolated from Gogi has been shown to have some anti-cancer effects. It also exhibits some immune enhancing properties. Gogi seems to be able to act as a radiosensitizer in mice. In another study, seventy-nine patients with advanced cancer, enrolled in a trial in which they were treated with lymphocyte-activated killer cells + interleukin-2, and some of the patients also received polysaccharides from Lycium barbarum. The patients that received Gogi showed a 41 percent response rate compared to 16 percent in those who did not receive the Gogi polysaccharides.

Grape Cure

is based on a simple diet and was discovered in the 1920's by **Johanna Brandt**. It relies on the strong affinity of cancer for glucose to help cancer cells ingest substances that are harmful to the cancer cells. The diet is basically a 12-hour fast followed by eating only concord (dark purple) grapes. Since the grapes contain resveratrol, pterostilbene, laetrile, ellagic acid, quercetin , cryptoxanthin and other carotenoids, and many other antioxidants, it is not surprising that this diet would have positive effects. While it may be noted that the diet includes lots of sugar, it is the idea that the sugar causes the cancer cells to take in other molecules that it normally would resist. The grapes are eaten slowly and continuously over 12 hours and then water fasting with non-chlorinated water, is practiced for the next 12 hours. Do not drink distilled water. The fasting part may be the most beneficial as it starves the cancer for several hours a day. This method should not be followed with pancreatic cancer, brain cancer, or bone cancer. While it is possible to substitute a combination of carrot and beet juice, do not combine the two remedies. Do not take large amounts of the grape diet. You want to starve the cancer cells as much as possible but feed them just enough of the mentioned anti-oxidants to cause them to die.

Grape seed extract (GSE)

contains highly concentrated polyphenols, which are also in grape juice and wine but in lower concentrations. The seeds also contain oligomeric proanthocyanidins, Vitamin E, linoleic acid, and flavinoids. GSE is well known as an anti-inflammatory. It has been shown to stop the growth of some cancers in culture. A recent study has shown that GSE does kill Leukemia cells in vitro. Another in vivo study showed a 59 to 73 percent inhibition of prostate tumor growth and a 47 percent reduction in tumor size. In the same study, it was shown that GSE strongly inhibited VEGF by 47 to 70 percent and at the same time, increased IGFBP-3 (insulin-like growth factor binding protein) by as much as 6 or 7 times. Levels of IGFBP-3 are a strong reverse indicator of prognosis.

Graviola

is a tree that grows in tropical South America and is related to the Paw-paw tree of North America. Its action is similar but reputed to be not as strong or effective by some. Graviola contains numerous acetogenins and is believed to inhibit ATP production in cancer cells.

Green Tea

contains a number of COX-2 inhibitors. Drink 5-10 cups daily or take the equivalent in capsules, natural is better. Epigallocatechin gallate (EGCG) and epigallocatechin (EGC) are similar to other flavinoids found in some brassicas and grapes that are known to kill cancer cells.

Herb Robert

sometimes used for diarrhea, to improve functioning of the liver and gallbladder, to reduce inflammation of the kidney, bladder, and gallbladder, and to prevent the formation of stones in the kidney, bladder, or gallbladder. Also used in some cases for cancer.

Horsetail

it has been found that horsetail halted the proliferation of cancer cells in some cases. A blend of herbs that included horsetail along with the mushroom chaga was effective at reducing lymphoma and leukemia tumors in some cases.

Hydrazine sulfate

is reported by some to be a very effective in reducing cachexia but should be used with care. Since it is a MAOI (monamine oxidase inhibitor), it may cause serious problems if mixed with some drugs or foods.

Hydrogen Peroxide

is reputed to be beneficial in fighting several cancers, especially lung cancer. A food-grade peroxide is required and may be taken by IV (administered by a medical professional), bathing in it, or it may be inhaled from a vaporizer.

Hypericum

(St. Johns Wort) has been used as a mood modulator. It has had many other suggested medicinal uses. Recent testing has shown that it kills certain lines of cancer cells.

Ibuprofen

is a NSAID and can cause stomach irritation as well as bleeding. It can also impair kidney function, especially in those who already have kidney problems. Ibuprofen reduces blood flow to the kidneys, which can aggravate congestive heart problems.

Indole-3-carbinol (I3C)

is a natural phytochemical isolated from cruciferous vegetables such as broccoli and Brussels sprouts that is effective in reducing certain hormone levels that influence cancer growth in some cancers such as breast cancer. I3C has been shown to stop cancer growth in some cases and induce cell death (apoptosis) in others. It has also been shown to be more effective than tamoxifen in inhibiting tumor cell growth in some cancer tests.

Inositol (Vitamin B11)

Activates NK cells.

Inositol hexaphosphate (IP-6)

activates NK cells, decreases cell proliferation, promotes normalization of cancer cells, and increases activity of the p53 tumor suppressor gene.

Insulin Potentiation Therapy

is the use of insulin to help transport drugs across cell membranes and even across the blood brain barrier more efficiently. Cancer cells generally have far more insulin receptors than normal cells, which makes them more sensitive to insulin. Shortly after the insulin injection, drugs and glucose are added. The basic results of IPT are increased permeability of tissues, including cell membranes and the blood brain barrier, metabolic changes in tumor cells, changes in blood chemistry, and changes in immune response. It is still chemotherapy.

Iodine

deficiency is suspected in gastric cancer, notable in certain areas where iodine ingestion is low. Iodine deficiency is also related to thyroid cancer. It is expected by some that iodine deficiency may play an even stronger role in cancer and in cancer healing. Many people have iodine deficiency so iodine should be included in any cancer therapy. The simplest way to test for iodine requirements is to paint the soft areas of the bottom of the feet with a known amount of Lugol's Iodine solution. One drop contains approx. 7.5 mg of elemental iodine and normal amounts are 4 to 6 drops spread evenly on each foot before bedtime. The body will only absorb the amounts needed, so that if some stain is still present upon wakening in the morning, the amount applied the next night can be reduced. If the stain is gone, continue painting iodine nightly until there is stain remaining in the morning. After this, reduce the amount of iodine used. This method has been safely in use for over 100 years.

Iron

is needed by cancer in order to grow. Check the blood chemistry. If the iron levels are above 100, bleeding or donating blood for research can reduce it. Caution; do not donate blood for transfusion because it may contain metastatic cancer cells. Also, lactoferrin may be beneficial in reducing iron content.

Japanese Knotweed

This edible plant contains vitamins and minerals and has been used in traditional medicine for centuries and in traditional Chinese medicine it is known as hu zhang, used to treat coughs, hepatitis, jaundice, amenorrhea, leukorrhea, arthralgia, and burns, as well as snake bites. It is also attested to be antiviral, antimicrobial, anti-inflammatory, neuroprotective, and exhibits cardioprotective abilities. Japanese knotweed contains high amounts of resveratrol.

Lactoferrin

deprives cancer cells of needed iron and inhibits angiogenesis. It is a glycoprotein that has been shown to have antibacterial, antiviral, anti-fungal, antioxidant, and anti-inflammatory properties. One of a group of substances known as cytokines, it may also be an immune modulator as there are receptor sites for lactoferrin on monocytes, lymphocytes, and neutrophils. A deficit of cytokines can lead to immunosuppression. Lactoferrin has been demonstrated as a major immune modulator in many circumstances and can reduce the death rate from septic shock significantly.

Laetrile

is often referred to as Vitamin B17 and has been a favorite anti cancer agent since the 1970s. It was initially proposed for its anti-cancer properties by Dr. Ernst T. Krebs. It is a nitriloside and enzymes (beta-glucosidase) that are only present in tumor cells reportedly releases cyanide in reaction to these enzymes, causing cell death in cancers. When B17 is introduced to the body, in normal cells, it is broken down by the enzyme Rhodanese into Thiocyanate and Benzoic acid which are beneficial to normal cellular metabolism. Mung bean sprouts, apricot kernels, almonds, apple seeds, and raw Macadamia nuts are good sources. Some cases of slight cyanide poisoning have been reported. You should expect more cyanide to be produced when large tumors are present. It would be a good idea to keep oxygen on hand and some anti-cyanide agents as an antidote such as hydroxycobalamin can be beneficial, converting to vitamin B-12 which may be used or excreted. Cimetidine (Tagamet) may reportedly serve the same purpose as Laetrile. There are several existing ethnic cultures that consume large amounts of nitrilosides and all are either free of cancer or have extremely low occurrence of cancer. Among these are the Hunzi, Eskimo, Hopi, Navaho, and the Abkahzians. Some want to claim that the cyanide containing substances are deadly, but then we would all be dead as the most common form of vitamin B12 is cyanocobalamin and strawberries also contain cyanide bearing compounds. As mentioned in the section on Amygdalin, there are some reported deaths from Laetrile ingestion, but there are some overlooked factors involved. Cyanide can be produced in the intestine if the cyanogenic glycosides are allowed to become alkaline. Be sensible when eating seeds containing Laetrile, according to some logic, if you eat three apples a day, the seeds in the three apples are sufficient B-17. You would not eat a pound of apple seeds. The same is true of peach seeds, apricot seeds, etc. and one peach or apricot kernel per 10 lbs of body weight is believed to be more than sufficient. Do not eat them with other foods and definitely do not take anything alkalizing with them. Eat a small amount, wait a while, the try a little more. Important: See cyanogenic glycosides

LDN

see Naltrexone, a Low Dose Naltrexone therapy.

Lycopene

is a carotenoid found in tomatoes that is especially effective in reducing prostate cancer in men. It may also be beneficial in reducing other cancers. Men who eat significant amounts of cooked tomatoes have about 80 percent less likelihood of developing prostate cancer.

is extremely important in both reducing the risk of cancer and in the effort to stop it. Actually, magnesium deficiency has been cited as a precursor to cancer as well as an indicator of cancer presence. In certain areas around the world, there are much higher amounts of magnesium in the water. In those areas, cancer occurs only a tenth as frequently or even less. There are other areas where magnesium is in very low supply and cancer occurs more frequently in those areas. You should get an absolute minimum of 500-mg magnesium in your diet and 3 to 3.5 grams a day will almost certainly significantly reduce any risk of getting cancer or many other illnesses as well. Magnesium should also be balanced with calcium, potassium, and sodium. Magnesium chloride is the preferred and most active source. Additionally, other alkaline minerals such as calcium, cesium, rubidium, and palladium will be beneficial. See **Epsom Salt**.

Mangosteen

is a tropical fruit with a purple colored outer shell, which is loaded with astringent phytochemicals and antioxidants. The astringents are effective against certain bacteria and fungi. While it is touted as a cancer cure, I have not seen any human studies to support this. There have been several studies indicating that compounds extracted from the bitter outer shell do have anticancer effects. However, much of the commercially available juice is made from that edible inner pulp which is low in antioxidants.

Mannitol

has been used to reduce intracranial pressure in cases of brain cancer. It also is used to open up the blood brain barrier.

Mannoheptulose

is a naturally occurring sugar that functions as a glucokinase inhibitor that reduces glucose uptake in cancer cells. It has been shown to reduce the growth rate in some human tumors in experimental animals.

Melatonin

is a natural hormone that modulates the immune system, helps restore restful natural sleep, improves normal blood cell production, and increases the effectiveness of IL-2 in tumor treatment. It is suggested that all cancer patients take from 15 mg to 20 mg of Melatonin nightly unless other medication suggests otherwise. Some sources recommend up to 40 mg nightly and dosages of up to 70 mg have been shown to be safe. It provides a natural sleep with no known side effects such as drowsiness. The use of **melatonin can increase the one-year survival rate from 2 to 40 times in certain cancers**. Most of the bodies healing and repair takes place during REM sleep and since REM sleep is the time at which the immune system is most active, one of the most important aspects of melatonin is that it increases REM sleep. Extremely high doses of melatonin (50 mg) dramatically increased REM sleep time and dream activity . Night workers have a significantly higher rate of cancer than those who sleep at night. Melatonin also regulates leptin which is reduced by higher concentrations of melatonin. In addition to being a powerful antioxidant, Melatonin is a direct scavenger of OH, O2$^-$, and NO. This allows it to reduce peroxides which are extremely damaging. In some studies, melatonin has singularly increased the life span of mice by 20 percent. I strongly suggest taking melatonin even if you do not have cancer but are over 40 years old. Taking very large amounts of melatonin can also have an effect as birth control because melatonin reduces Follicle Stimulating Hormone (FSH). In regards to toxicity, in rats, the no observable adverse effect level was 100 mg/kg/day. Translated to humans, this could be the equivalent of 7 grams a day for a person weighing 160 lbs but these levels are definitely not advised.

Metformin

has been used for over 20 years to treat diabetes in Canada and Europe but has been limited by the FDA in the US to Diabetics who can not take insulin. It has been shown to stop the development of pancreatic cancer in hamsters.

Methylsulfonylmethane (MSM)

is a sulfur-based compound that is related to DMSO. It is reputed as a pain reliever and anti-inflammatory and is used in arthritis, fibromyalgia, and gout. Some studies have indicated that MSM may induce differentiation in certain cancer cell lines, causing an end to proliferation. MSM is actually a triple whammy to cancer. First, it is a methylator as it contributes a methyl radical to help support methylation. Second, it is sulfur base and provides sulfur for many processes. Third, is provides a concentrated source of the essential amino acid , methionine that is critical for the proper functioning of cellular metabolism.

MGN-3

is a rice bran extract that has been shown to increase the number of NK cells circulating in the blood. It is assumed that the increased NK cells will attack cancer cells. No research could be found to verify any cancer reduction.

Milk Thistle

has been used for thousands of years to help heal. It is especially well known for its ability to remove toxins and heal the liver. It is even used as an antidote for Amanita mushroom which is considered to be deadly. Milk Thistle is a naturally growing wild herb that is also sometimes combined with NAC (n-Acetyl Cysteine) and ALA (alpha Lipoic Acid) for helping with liver regeneration.

Mistletoe

contains viscotoxins, which are obtained from extracts and increase cytotoxicity associated with NK cell activity in some European studies.

Modified Citrus Pectin (MCP)

reduces cancer growth and metastasis. It is thought to prevent metastasis by blocking the ability of cancers to bind to other cells. Consider taking this before any biopsy as biopsies are a cause of cancer metastasis and spread.

is one substance that while it does not stop or reduce cancer, it does stop the pain. The reason that I am adding morphine to the list is as a warning. Once the pain of cancer is so great that only morphine will work, there may not much that can be done except to keep the patient comfortable. Once a cancer sufferer is on morphine they may lose their desire to drink or take nutrition. Organ function may be impaired. The bowels and kidneys may not function as well as they should. There may be little motivation for life left.

Mustard

is a brassica and is available in various forms, from mustard greens to prepared yellow mustard. Mustard contains significant amounts of glucosinolates such as isothiocyanates and thiocyanates, which have anti-cancer properties.

N-acetyl-cysteine (NAC)

is a powerful antioxidant, anti-carcinogenic, and anti-mutagenic agent. It also inhibits angiogenesis. Helps reduce or avoid liver damage from some drugs such as acetaminophen. It is often used as a chelator of heavy metals such as mercury. NAC may also have a negative effect on insulin receptors. It is important in protecting the liver, kidneys, and other organs from damage. Cysteine is an essential amino acid that is important in many cellular functions. Many cancer patients are found to be low in cysteine and in some studies, individuals with low cysteine have a much higher risk of developing cancer. Those who have high levels of cysteine have little risk of developing cancer.

Cysteine is also a precursor to glutathione which is also extremely important.

Naltrexone

when taken in low dosages may cause cancers to shrink and go into remission but this effect only lasts while the low dose naltrexone is being taken. Naltrexone is legal and according to several sources, normal dosage is 3 mg nightly at bedtime. The use of naltrexone can buy time for other therapies to work.

Neem

has been found to increase white blood cell counts in many cases. It has been used for centuries in Southeast Asia to reduce tumors. According to recent studies, neem contains a group of polysaccharides and limonoids that inhibits cancer cell adhesion. The salve or ointment appears to be effective against skin cancers. In some cases, it is effective in reducing diabetes, cholesterol, and high blood pressure.

Niacin

is a water soluble vitamin (B3) that is important in a number of body functions. See: Vitamin B3.

Nitrilosides

See amygdalin:

Noni juice

has been shown to reduce angiogenesis in tumors and in large concentrations may even cause degeneration in existing vessels. Noni may also be effective in preventing the formation of cancerous cells. It is high in anti-oxidants and this may partially explain some of its effects. It is also high in sugars, which can possibly have a negative effect. Additionally, because sugars stimulate digestive juices and enzymes, which destroy the active products in Noni, most Noni juice is not effective. If you take Noni, it should be fresh and should not be sweet for maximum effectiveness.

Oleander

has been used medicinally as far back as 3500 years ago and as a cancer treatment as far back as 1000 years ago. A patented extract of Oleander, Anvirzel has passed FDA phase 1 trials. Oleander is **highly toxic in its raw form** and can be lethal if not properly prepared. It should not be handled with bare hands. It has been shown to be a powerful immune stimulator. There are several sites on the Internet that provide additional information and instructions on how to safely prepare oleander soup.

Omega-3 fatty acids

have been shown to reduce the occurrence of prostate, ovarian, pancreatic, and breast cancers. They are known to be anti-inflammatory in nature and counteract Omega-6 fatty acids. Alpha linolenic acid when ingested is converted by the body to EPA and DHA. Alpha linolenic acid is common in flax seed oil, which is a major part of the Budwig protocol for cancer treatment. In cases where cachexia is present, 2 grams of EPA is recommended daily. See DHA, EPA, Fish oil, arachadonic acid, ALA (alpha-linoleic acid) are PUFAs and are generally considered as inflammatory and should be reduced in general. Omega-6 is common in corn oil, sunflower oil, dairy products, and meats. The proposed ideal dietary ratio is 1 omega-3 to 4 omega-6. The normal U.S. diet is about 1:16 due to high red meat content as well as the use of corn oil vs olive oil for food preparation. See Arachodonic acid, Omega-3 fatty acids

Omega-9 fatty acids

is found in olives, olive oil, avocados, almonds, peanuts, and pecans. It is not considered essential as the body can manufacture these products.

Onion

has been shown to reduce the risk of cancer and the more pungent the better according to some. Onions contain the compound quercetin, which has been shown to reduce certain cancers. Onions also contain allyl propyl disulphide and other sulfur based compounds, which give onion much of its flavor and may also, benefit cancer reduction.

Oregano

the essential oil of Oregano contains 4-terpineol which is effective against the spread of cancer in some cancers but not others.

Oxygen

is important in battling cancer because cancer thrives in an oxygen poor environment. Some cancer sufferers spend time in hyperbaric oxygen chambers and others try to boost their oxygen levels by drinking or bathing in hydrogen peroxide. Food grade (35%) hydrogen peroxide is often used, and for bathing, 8 ounces is added to a filled tub of bath water. For placing into a humidifier, 1 ounce is placed into a gallon of water. In some cases, patients are given hydrogen peroxide by IV injection.

Ozone

is used to boost oxygen levels in some cases and the most common methods are infusion and Ozone IV therapy. In ozone infusion, some blood is removed from the body and is infused with ozone and replaced. Ozone therapies are used everywhere in the world except in the US. There are no studies showing that it does not work and many showing that it does. The FDA has blocked all attempts at having tests conducted in the US.

Ozone IV Therapy

adds additional oxygen to the blood by injecting a solution of ozone into the bloodstream.

Pancreatic enzymes

taken in large doses by patients with pancreatic cancer can greatly extend life expectancy. This therapy is now being investigated by the NCI. Traditionally, pancreatic enzymes were considered as purely digestive in nature. While this aspect is true, these enzymes can digest proteins both in the digestive system and in the body as well. If a person eats significant amounts of meats and other protein sources, the available supply of pancreatin is consumed for digestion of these proteins, leaving insufficient amounts for internal use. If a person eats late night meals, then this continues to reduce the amount of pancreatin available. Generally, it appears to take roughly 12 hours after eating a significant amount of protein for the body to recover its pancreatin levels so that it can use it internally. The importance of this in relation to cancer is that cancer cells have cell membranes that are up to 15 times thicker than normal cell membranes and they have higher than normal amounts of protein in their cell membranes and pancreatin can digest these proteins, killing the cancer cells. This is also probably just one reason why the fasting therapies have benefit in fighting cancer. Things that are incompatible with pancreatic enzymes are alcohols, including sugar alcohols, and low pH (acidic condition). There are a lot of cancer sufferers who have benefited from the Kelley / Gonzales therapies, which utilize pancreatin combined with other protocols. Some individuals have taken as much as 60 grams of pancreatin daily.

Papaya

is a fruit, which is rich in papain, a protease enzyme that can help break down the protein coating that cancer cells often use for protection from the immune system.

Parthenolide

is an active anti-cancer compound found in Feverfew. It has been shown as effective in causing apoptosis in cases of AML (acute myelogenous leukemia). It has also been shown to inhibit growth in pancreatic cell lines and to increase apoptosis in other tumor cells.

has been known to be fairly high in anti-oxidants, however, it also inhibits both the proliferation and migration of cancer cells in the body.

has been shown in scientific studies to have pain killing, anti-inflammatory, and anti-cancer abilities. It is available as a dried bark for teas and as an extract. It contains chemicals known as naphthaquinones that are thought to enhance the immune system.

is an ATP inhibitor that is preferentially absorbed by active cancer cells and interferes with mitochondrial and cellular regulation processes. Not recommended to be used with CoQ10, or antioxidants. The Pawpaw tree is native to the eastern U.S. and extracts have been sold in the U.S. since the late 1800's. Prior to that time, American Indians used Pawpaw for many years.

At least three acetogenic compounds, bullatacin, asimicin, and trilobacin have been identified in Pawpaw extract.

is the natural source of capsaicin, piperine, piperidine, and other substances known to help fight cancers. In countries that consume large amounts of spicy peppers, there tends to be a lower incidence of cancer. See **Habanero**:

Phenethyl isothiocyanate

is a compound found in cruciferous vegetables such as broccoli that has been shown to inhibit EGFR, a hormone that spurs the growth of ovarian cancers.

Phycotene

is a combination of carotenoids extracted from spirulina and dunaliella that can not only protect from cancer but also may even reverse it. It has been shown to activate Interleukin, enhance the immune response, and increases the amount of tumor necrosis factor that is available from macrophages to kill cancer cells.

Piperine

is an important alkaloid, responsible for the punch of black pepper, that modulates enzyme activities and improves the absorption of certain substances such as curcumin and selenium. It inhibits angiogenesis and also increases the serum levels of some substances such as co-enzyme Q10 and B-carotene.

Plantain

which is a weed found growing in many yards, has been found to strongly suppress the growth of human cancer cells.

Poly-MVA

is a combination of alpha lipoic acid, vitamins, minerals, and amino acids with palladium. It has shown impressive results in terminally ill cancer patients. It is reported that some hospice patients recovered and were able to walk out on their own. Poly-MVA can pass through the blood brain barrier because it is both, water soluble and fat soluble, providing new hope for those with brain tumors. There are no known side effects, however for it to be most effective, reduce all antioxidants to a minimum.

Pomegranate

fruit contains a large number of antioxidants, which makes it beneficial in reducing cancer and its effects. Many juices are available but the best are fresh, not pasteurized, and kept refrigerated.

Potassium

is one of the most important minerals that the body needs. It is essential for normal good health and function of the circulatory system, nervous system, kidneys, and cellular metabolism. It is also one mineral that many people do not get enough of. Potassium is available from many foods in small amounts. If needed in larger amounts, it is in the grocery store as "No Salt" and is also combined with sodium as "Morton Lite". It is important to balance sodium and potassium. Almost everything excreted by the kidneys requires potassium.

Probiotics

are critical in the maintenance of good health and are very important in fighting cancer. The first thing to know is that vegetable fiber is very important in maintaining proper beneficial bacteria in the intestine. Probiotics produce beneficial short chain fatty acids in the intestine and reduce certain carcinogenic enzymes.

are powerful in that they inhibit functions such as viral replication. They are often used to help fight HIV. Some cancers are also caused by viral infections.

Protocell

See Cancell.

Quercetin

is a flavonol found in many medicinal plants and is anti-inflammatory. It also has a number of anti-tumor properties as it blocks NF-κB. High levels of quercetin may be found in capers and lovage. It is also present in onions.

Raw foods

contain enzymes and other active proteins that are destroyed by cooking or heating food. Many people suspect that the elimination or reduction of raw foods from the diet is a major cause of cancer. It is certainly known that some of the enzymes obtained from raw foods are helpful in preventing aging.

Red clover

contains genistein, which is a vascular growth inhibitor. It inhibits the development of new blood vessels in tumors, which slows their growth. It is also high in isoflavones and has been used for centuries as a blood purifier. Do not use red clover if your are taking estrogen, progesterone, tamoxiphen, or have cancers that have estrogen positive receptors such as breast or uterine cancer. Red clover can also interfere with certain blood thinners.

are reported to have powerful antioxidant properties that can enhance the body's immune response. They also contain complex sugars known as beta-glucans that are believed to stop the growth of cancer cells and reduce metastasis. They have also been linked to reduced blood pressure, improved nerve function, and greater stamina.

Resveratrol

shows antimutagenic, anti-inflammatory, and antioxidant properties. It also functions as a COX-2 inhibitor and has anticancer effects

Rhubarb

contains an ingredient that speedily kills cancer in 48 hours. According to some reports it destroyed the cancer but left healthy blood cells unscathed. A derivative, called S3, slashed the growth of lung cancer by a factor of three in just 11 days, tests on mice showed. The same effect was seen on cells from head and neck tumors.

Selenium

helps activate some important antioxidants, facilitates DNA repair, and causes apoptosis or cell death in some cancers. Supplementation with 200 mcg daily can significantly reduce mortality from cancers.

Serotonin

has been found to be a key driver in stimulating a natural cell "suicide" process for controlling the runaway growth that leads to cancer. Certain anti-depressants such as Paxil, Prozac, and other **SSRIs prevented serotonin from being absorbed into the cancer cells,** leading to a more vigorous growth of tumors in vitro. Researchers in Canada found that Tamoxafen combined with paroxetine increased the mortality risk in breast cancer patients and that the longer the two therapies were combined together, the greater the mortality. Another study from the Univ. of Cincinatti shows that breast cancer cells produce serotonin and that the breast cancer cells also have serotonin receptor sites that do not function normally and contribute to abnormal cell growth.

Serrapeptase or *wobenzyme*

enzyme is a fibrinolytic enzyme that attacks fibrin which is a protein coating that cancer cells and tumors use to cloak and protect their surface. These enzymes have been used in Europe for over 30 years.

Shark cartilage

has been promoted for cancer on the basis that sharks have survived for millions of years and rarely get cancer. Regardless of the reason, a lot of individuals have experienced positive results from taking shark cartilage.

Shark Liver Oil

helps boost the immune system, reduces anemia, and helps prevent angiogenesis. A major constituent of shark liver oil is alkylglycerols, which stimulate white blood cells, macrophages, as well as the production of cytokines. The results are anti-fungal and anti-bacterial. Shark liver oil also contains squalene, Vitamins A,D, omega-3 fatty acids, glycol ethers, and fatty alcohols.

Silibinin

is extracted from milk thistle, functions as an antioxidant and inhibits the COX-2 enzyme. It also serves to protect the liver and is considered effective in fighting almost every type of liver disease.

slippery elm

has been used for centuries, the soft inner bark of the slippery elm tree (Ulmus fulva) has been used by Native Americans for treatment in a variety of health conditions, including: Skin wounds and burns, Sore throat, Cough, and Acid Reflux/Heartburn as well as Inflammatory Bowel Disease. It is used in **Essiac Tea:**

Sodium bicarbonate

injections have been shown to have a significant effect in reducing cancers. A 5 percent solution of sodium bicarbonate is injected into the body, thereby raising the blood pH and causing significant tumor reduction. This strongly supports the acid-alkaline theory of cancer origin and treatment. See: Simoncini, Bicarbonate of Soda

sheep sorrel

is another herb that is used in **Essiac Tea**. As it is the main cancer killing agent in Essiac, it has been known for its cancer fighting properties for over 100 years. ***Soy***

protein extract contains several compounds including genistein that are helpful in fighting cancer. Because of the presence of certain amino acids, soy protein should not be used with hydrazine sulfate. Normally breast cancer patients should avoid soy products as certain breast cancer cells may proliferate faster when genistein is absorbed.

Spirulina

is a cyanobacteria that has significant nutritional value. It is protein rich, rich in omega fatty acids, loaded with vitamins, powerful antioxidants, and is loaded with alkalizing minerals. Spirulina grows as mats of bacteria in pools of warm water and has been produced in tropical climates for over 1000 years. There have been a number of studies showing that spirulina can boost immune function. It is even stated that spirulina should not be taken in cases of over active immune systems such as with lupus. Another expressed concern is that spirulina has significant concentrations of minerals that may build up excessively with long term consumption.

SSRIs

serotonin re-uptake inhibitors such as Prozac, Paxil and Celexa, encouraged growth of a type of cancer called Burkitt's lymphoma in the test tube.

Theanine

is a free amino acid that is found in tea leaves and works to create a state of relaxation. It also helps to fight cancer in several ways. It is a glutamate substitute that causes the production of defective glutathione. The altered glutathione does not protect cancer cells as normal glutathione does.

Trypsin

is a proteolytic enzyme that may help remove the protective protein coat from certain cancer cells.

Tryptophan

is an essential amino acid and a precursor for several important hormones including serotonin, melatonin, and for the vitamin B3, niacin.

Thymus extract

can help boost immune function, especially in individuals over 40 years old and in those whose immune system is impaired.

Ukrain

is extracted from a weed and has been found to be very effective against some pancreatic cancers and others. Clinical studies indicate that it may be effective against several cancer types. In a study on colorectal cancer, Ukrain was found to have more than twice the two-year survival rate when compared to 5-flourouracil and radiation.

Urea

has a double relationship in regards to cancer. First, it is an important biological indicator in reference to kidney function. BUN (blood urea nitrogen) is an indicator for kidney activity. Additionally, urea has anticancer properties, especially when injected around tumor sites of certain types of cancers. Orally ingested urea has been shown to extend life in some liver cancers, cause remission in others, and also shows benefit in small metastatic lung tumors.

Vitamin A

is particularly important in fighting cancer, especially as an immune system booster and as an antioxidant. It should be noted that there is a strong link with vitamin A deficiency and the development of cancer in some cases. Vitamin A is particularly important during radiation therapy as it helps avoid some of the damage to normal cells. Some oncologists, however, believe that vitamin A interferes with the effects of radiation on the cancer. However, it can be helpful in reducing damage to normal cells during radiation. Also, it should be noted that vitamin A might be only one of several similar substances known as carotenoids that combine for maximum results. Good sources are carrots and cod liver oil. See Carotenoids.

Vitamin B1or Thiamine

has been shown to help relieve pain associated with nerves such as neuritis and neuropathy. It has been shown in studies with rats, but not human studies, that excess thiamine supports the growth of some cancers. The main problem is that cancer cells produce ribose (a 5 carbon sugar that is the base of DNA) in a process that uses thiamine instead of the ribose production process that is used by normal cells which requires oxygen. Cancer cells must produce DNA in order to replicate. On the other hand, thiamine is essential in proper amounts to prevent the buildup of lactic acid in the blood of cancer patients

.Vitamin B2 or Riboflavin

has been linked to mood and may be beneficial in reducing depression associated with cancer. It is also well known that riboflavin deficiencies as directly linked to certain conditions of poor health because it is important in the metabolism regulation of iron, and can lead to anemia when iron intakes are low. It is interesting that riboflavin deficiency can develop fairly rapidly indicating a need for constant replacement or the lack of reserves, especially since riboflavin is a water soluble vitamin. It is also noted that a deficiency of riboflavin may contribute to a reduced metabolism of folic acid and pyridoxine. It is a precursor to its most important biologically active forms, flavin adenine dinucleotide (FAD) and flavin mononucleotide (FMN), which are involved in a number of processes that are critical to the function of aerobic cells. That aside, some studies indicate that riboflavin deficiency inhibits the growth of several tumors but the exact mechanisms have not yet been determined. In some other cases, such as azo dye induced tumors of the liver are increased when a deficiency of riboflavin is present. Riboflavin also influences the uptake of the drug methotrexate by neoplastic cells. Foods that contribute the most riboflavin are milk and other dairy products. Fish and dark green vegetables also contribute some

.Vitamin B3 or Niacin

is important in normal body processes and helps prevent or reduce cancer. It is also associated with relieving depression and anxiety. It helps maintain proper cholesterol levels in the blood, increasing HDL. The best form of Niacin is the nicotinic acid (B3) form and not the hexanicotinate (flush free) form. A niacin flush is an indicator that it is working. A timed-release form can help reduce but not eliminate the flush, however, this form may cause liver toxicity. The flush is a result of releasing histamines, which if the immune system is in proper condition will result in antagonism toward cancer cells. Niacin expands the capillaries, which allows histamines to exit cells where they have been stored. It also is important in the generation of serotonin. Another important aspect of Niacin is that it is involved in a significant portion of the electron transfer that takes place in the formation of ATP. Much of the electon transfer is through NAD (Nicotine Adenine Dinucleotide) and NADP, the phosphate bearing form of the same. Both are derivatives of Nicotinic acid. A shortage of Nicotinic acid may cause a reduction in the amount of NAD and NADP available thereby reducing cellular energy. The body can produce limited amounts of Niacin through the conversion of tryptophan, but it is done at the expense of considerable cellular energy. Any excess Niacin can be excreted in the urine. It is very low in toxicity and may be extremely beneficial. In one study, participants who took 3 grams of full flush Niacin a day over 10 years experienced a 90 percent reduction in mortality and occurrence of heart attacks as well as a significant reduction in the occurrence of cancers. Full flush Niacin may cause serious flushes when first taken and these flushes may last from 10 minutes to over an hour. Flushes tend to reduce in extent over continued use.

is active in the formation of some hormones and is also important in wound healing. It is also an adrenal activator and may be helpful in reducing fatigue.

helps reduce homocysteine levels and has been shown to offer protection against certain cancers. Three forms of B6, pyridoxine, pyridoxal, and pyridoxamine are precursors of an activated compound known as <u>pyridoxal 5'-phosphate</u> (PLP), which plays a vital role as the cofactor of a large number of essential enzymes in the human body. It is extremely important for a properly functioning immune system. Vitamin B6 may in some cases improve the long-term effectiveness of some pain relievers and can also reduce inflammation. It is important not to take vitamin B6 without other B vitamins.

Vitamin B12

is available as cyanocobalamin or methylcobalamin and is an important co-enzyme that helps reduce homocysteine levels by the process of methylation. Low levels of B12 have been associated with pernicious anemia. Vitamin B12 in large doses can also provide significant pain relief in some cases. Methylcobalamin is more easily absorbed and can more easily cross the blood brain barrier than cyanocobalamin can, therefore, it should be the form used when B-12 is taken. Methylcobalamin is also a contributor to the methylation process which makes it even more important. An excess methylcobalamin will be safely excreted in the urine.

Vitamin C

enhances immune function and is a strong antioxidant. It has the ability in some cases to stop or limit the spread of cancers and in others has shown the ability to eliminate tumors altogether. It has been shown to be able to reduce angiogenesis in many tumors. Large dosages of vitamin C are safe but if taken orally, it can cause diarrhea. Many cancer sufferers take from 10 to 15 grams a day orally while some others take up to 100 grams daily intravenously. Adding vitamin B-12, selenium, and Alpha Lipoic Acid can increase the efficiency of Vitamin C. As with other therapies, increase dosages gradually. Vitamin C also has been noted to reduce pain in some cases.

Vitamin C IV

when given by intravenous injection, vitamin C can reach much higher levels in the blood and body. This has been shown to produce dramatic improvements in many cases.

Vitamin D

is normally formed in the skin as a result of exposure to sunlight. It is significantly involved in the regulation of calcium absorption by cells in the body. There is also a strong correlation between certain cancers such as breast cancer, colon cancer, and intestinal cancer and the amount of sunlight exposure available. Cancer therapy doses range from 1800 IU to 3000 IU or more, even 8000 IU to 10000 IU for limited periods of time. If the dosage exceeds 3000 IU daily, it is important to monitor liver and kidney function on a monthly basis using standard CBC blood chemistry tests.

Vitamin E

is a powerful antioxidant that can inhibit many cancers, protect against the effects of radiation therapy, and improve the results of some other therapies. It is important to use gamma-tocopherol as well as alpha-tocopherol. It is actually the gamma-tocopherol that is most important as it neutralizes peroxynitrite, a major free radical. Cancer patients will often take 400 IU to 1200 IU daily of mixed tocopherols and tocotrienols.

Vitamin K1

This used to be the standard form of vitamin K and is responsible for the clotting of blood among other things. The important thing about K1 is that it needs to be properly in balance with vitamin K2.

Vitamin K2

also known as menaquinone which is found in animal foods and fermented foods such as Natto. It is also found in egg yolks. It interferes with the development and growth of some specific cancers in addition to being important for vascular health.

Wheat grass

may be harvested from young shoots and juiced to provide a wide range of antioxidants and enzymes. It is also considered to be a good alkalizer because of its mineral content.

Wild Lettuce

or Lactuca virosa, or opium lettuce, is a plant with psychoactive effects and can be found growing freely in various regions of the world including Australia, America, Southern Europe and India. While milder than morphine, wild lettuce has similar effects but does not have opiates in it. For this reason, it is legal to forage, to grow, and own without prescription or license.

Also known as Goji berry and Chinese wolfberry, it has been used for over 2000 years as a health tonic and to promote longevity, as a sexual stimulant, analgesic, and as an antibacterial. It has been shown to induce apoptosis in certain cancer cell lines.

porous aluminosilicate mineral found naturally in volcanic rock and ashes. It is known to cause some cancer when the dust is inhaled. Theoretically believed to absorb toxins, thereby helping remove them and reducing cancer.

Therapies and protocols

Bob Beck

His protocol consists of four parts that work together in helping the body heal itself.

Part 1 is known as Blood Electrification or Micropulsing. Using a micropulse pulse generator device with electrodes placed over the arteries in the wrist, on the ankle, or both, mild electrical currents pass through the skin, reaching the bloodstream. As the current passes through the bloodstream, it kills or destroys microbes as it passes through them. This type of device is known as a Beck Zapper or Bob Beck Blood Electrifier (BBBE). It was designed based on the work of Kaali and Lyman, and is not the same as a Hulda Clark Zapper although there are some similarities. I believe that it might be even more beneficial to add a good multi-frequency Clark Zapper when doing the Beck protocol.

Part 2 uses Pulsed Electro-Magnetic Fields (PEMF) to generate microcurrents of electromagnRadio frequencyetic energy for targeting specific areas of the body. This provides a way to disable harmful pathogens hiding in tissues and organs and other non-blood systems. PEMF is recognized to help alleviate joint and muscle pain due to injury or chronic arthritis, and can aid in the healing process of bone fractures, soft tissue injuries and sports injuries.

Part 3 is the use of colloidal silver which is safe and effective as a natural antibacterial, antiviral and anti-fungal, having been used in health care in various cultures for thousands of years. Silver can also help prevent and heal infections such as respiratory ailments and MRSA.

Part 4 involves drinking water enriched with ozone helps to increase the oxygen level in the body as well as assisting the breakdown and removal of toxins from the body.

Biopsy and Biopsies

I find it extremely sad that whenever someone appears to have some form of cancer, the first thing that a doctor wants to do is perform a biopsy, taking a sample of the suspect cancer to see if it is actually cancerous. Years back, when I had a cancerous lesion on my temple that I had determined to be basal cell skin cancer on my own, I had requested that the lesion be removed using mohs surgery. The doctor refused to do so stating that he had to do a biopsy first and the surgery would be done after determination that the biopsied sample was truly cancerous.

I was angry but went ahead. By the time that the results came back positive and the surgery was scheduled, the skin cancer had spread to 3 satellite lesions as a result of the biopsy. When the surgery was being done, I requested that these be removed at the same time. Again the doctor refused stating that a new biopsy would be required. After the surgery, I never returned and the doctor is still sending me urgent letters telling me that I need to get the cancers treated. It has been almost 13 years.

I never told the doctor that I used an alternative method and got rid of my cancers over the next few weeks. There was a couple of new lesions that popped up over the next months but I took care of them the same way.

This, however is not about how I treated my cancer but is about the abomination of using such a primitive, outdated procedure such as biopsy.

The real problem with performing a biopsy is that it opens the cancer up, allowing it to spread. Normally, especially where tumorous cancers are concerned, the cancer is walled off by the body, It is encased in an envelope to keep it from spreading. Once the encasement has been cut through the cancer cells can easily escape and migrate to other places in the body. This should never be allowed but continues because it is highly profitable. The doctor gets more money and the spread of cancer can really increase the financial outcome.

So, what is the alternative to biopsy?

For many cancers, thermographic imaging can quickly tell if there is an active cancer due to the heat being produced. For example, benign tumors do not produce any significant heat because they are not highly metabolic whereas cancerous tumors produce significant heat because they are very active. A thermographic imaging system can see this quickly and easily.

This can be more difficult for some deep internal cancers but today, we also have a number of tumor markers in the blood that we can analyze for such as VEGF, CEA, HCG, among many others.
The point of all this is that the medical industry needs to move forward and leave behind its highly antiquated diagnostics.

Brandt diet

book on the grape cure was published in the 1920s. Much has been learned since the 1920s and many things have changed. The original diet involves 12 hours of fasting every day, followed by 12 hours where you consume absolutely nothing except grapes (and/or grape juice).

Start the treatment like this:

Begin with a 24 oz. bottle of (dark concord) grape juice the first thing in the morning. Do not eat until Noon. Take a couple of swallows every 10 or 15 minutes (Don't gulp it down all at once).
After 12 o'clock, live the rest of the day normally, but do not eat anything after 8 o'clock in the evening...food seems to carry off the curative agent in the grape juice, which may be magnesium, so stick to the fast between 8 P.M. and Noon the following day.

Keep this up every day for 2 weeks to one month. I'd appreciate hearing of the firsthand results of this treatment. The more cases, the better the evidence.

Krebiozen is fine, but it racks up only about 80% cures, and is no longer available due to the federal injunction suit, the F.D.A., the A.M.A., etc. Ditto "Mucorihicin", the 87% effective cancer treatment from Pittsburgh. The dark concord grape juice treatment is reported to be nearly 100% effective.

Breuss Diet

The Breuss diet is based on a 42 day fast, but the definition of "fast" used in the Breuss diet actually includes certain types of foods, such as raw fruits and vegetable juices, all taken in liquid form. The theory is that cancer cells can only live on the protein of solid food. Therefore, if you drink nothing but vegetable juice and teas for 42 days the cancerous cells die while the normal cells continue to thrive. *Breuss juice vegetable juice that consists of 55 percent red beet root, 20 percent carrots, 20 percent celery root, 3 percent raw potato, 2 percent radishes ... If you look at the formula for the Breuss juice during the fast, you will note that there is virtually no glucose or other sugars in the formula.*

Budwig Protocol

Dr. Johanna Budwig was a leading researcher on oils and fats and their effects on the body. In her research, she discovered that many of the

conventional processed fats and hydrogenated oils were affecting our
cell membranes, contributing to defective cell membranes and
increasing diseased cells and toxicity.

As a result of her work, she created a diet that she claimed to have had
over a 90 percent success rate in fighting cancer over a 50-year period!

When you replace the processed fats and oils with
unsaturated/saturated fatty acids such as Omega-3s, your cells are able
to rebuild rejuvenate. She found that combining a mixture of cottage
cheese, flaxseeds, and flaxseed oil had the best results.

The sulfur protein rich cottage cheese and the flax are combined,
improving the ability to absorb these vital nutrients.

There are several different recipes available but I like this one.

Recipe:

6 tablespoons cold pressed flaxseed oil.

2/3 cup of organic low-fat cottage cheese.

Blend it with a blender for a couple of minutes until you get a
mixture where the oil doesn't separate from the cheese.

Add two tablespoons of fresh ground flax seed meal to the mixture.

½ cup of chopped nuts or organic berries.

Add some cinnamon.

Add water to make the mixture thinner if needed.

Use a spoon to stir the mixture if you want to make it thinner, but don't make it very thin.

You may also add:

3 to 4 tablespoons sprouted and ground chia or flax

1 teaspoon turmeric powder

1/4 teaspoon black pepper

Mix all the ingredients together in bowl or blender and consume once daily.

Sometimes in place of the nuts or berries, I will substitute apple sauce or peaches, which are probably not as beneficial, just help by adding variety.

Cellect-Budwig

This combination of two well known protocols may become effective within days. Although the protocol focuses on cancer treatment, it has also been found to be effective in many other chronic and terminal health issues.

The main part of this protocol is a nutritional powder called Cellect, which has shown excellent results with all forms of cancer and many other chronic or terminal health issues.

Additionally, The Budwig Diet is added to restore cellular integrity and the electrical charge in the cells.

Electromedicine has the ability to safely and quickly remove cancer cells from the body. It is also believed to shrink tumors, quickly in many cases, and it can reduce pain dramatically. This part of the protocol uses an expensive Rife machine that modulates with RF and uses a plasma tube. The setup costs several thousand dollars to procure.

Although highly suppressed, Laetrile or B17 has been a natural cancer treatment for several decades. It can selectively kill cancer cells safely, not so fast that it creates dangerous debris.

The addition of vegetable juicing is important for two major reasons. First, several included vegetables are high in anti-cancer nutrients. Secondly, focusing on vegetable juice allows you to crowd out the bad foods that most people eat

The protocol has a series of videos that the follower should watch as they can provide critical information that is not included here.

While today Dr. Clark is harassed and victimized by the pharmaceutical industry, the FDA, the FTC, and some other members of medical community under the guise of quackwatch and quackbusters, she is considered by many who have used her techniques and protocols to be a hero and will in the future be hailed for her efforts to forward modern medical thought. Her claims are a threat to the drug companies and to surgical hospitals which are the basis of health care throughout the world. The worldwide medical care system is about to suffer massive losses and is struggling to prevent this although almost everything that Dr. Clark claims is supported in current textbooks.

Just what are these claims that Dr. Clark makes? **Dr. Clark** claims that much of our bad health comes from chemicals and toxins that we are subjected to on a daily basis. Among these chemicals are mercury from amalgam dental fillings and isopropyl alcohol from cleaning products and many others. She also claims that in addition to these chemicals that there are many parasites that invade our bodies and cause illness. Her solution to the problem of health is to eliminate these foreign contaminations. Remove unwanted metals and chemicals from your body, eliminate disease causing parasites, drink water to keep your body cleaned out, eat proper chemical free and parasite free foods for nutrition. What could be simpler than a clean healthy diet and a clean healthy environment?

So what is wrong with her claims? First, the claim about mercury puts the American Dental Association in a bad position. They have been telling people for years that dental amalgam is safe. It is not! Once an amalgam filling has been placed in your mouth, it starts poisoning your body. The saliva in your mouth combined with enzymes secreted by bacteria leaches mercury from these fillings and you swallow it. Additionally, mercury vapors escape from the filling and you breath them in injuring your lungs and poisoning your blood. If you have any doubt about the toxicity of mercury, I can tell you. I once dropped a mercury thermometer in the chemistry lab. They evacuated the lab and the entire building until cleanup and decontamination was completed by people dressed up in hazard suits. The ADA has poisoned a majority of the people in this country with mercury and refuses to own up to its mistake despite the fact that European countries and others around the world now classify dental amalgam as hazardous and prohibit its use.

The second problem is with parasites causing cancer and other illness. Just pick up any good textbook on parasitology and read it. It will tell you that parasites cause cancer, intestinal disorders, liver and kidney failure, as well as many other illnesses. So why does the medical profession deny this? They will tell you that flukes mentioned by Dr. **Hulda Clark** exist only in Southeast Asia in order to debunk her theories. They are wrong! While many of these flukes are indigenous to SE Asia, they are not limited to that area. Many **soldiers from the Vietnam war unknowingly brought these parasites back with them** contaminating their families and others. Additionally, many **Americans travel to Thailand, Malaysia, Borneo, and Indonesia every year** and bring back more of these parasites. Because these parasites were not expected to appear in the US, the medical schools have taught the medical students (now doctors) not to bother looking for these parasites. You can look in third grade or fourth grade health books to find out about parasites but many doctors do not even acknowledge their existence.

The third problem is the stubbornness of the medical community. If a change does not make their job either easier or more profitable, the **doctors and the AMA do not want it**. Society is lead to believe that the AMA is there to promote good medical practices. It is not! **The primary function of the AMA is to preserve the income and status of its members**. The medical profession has cost us millions of lives of loved ones by refusing to accept change. This can be seen in the persistence of the idea of spontaneous generation which was perpetuated for hundreds of years. The idea was shown to be wrong in 1668 by Francesco Redi' but it took almost 200 years before the medical profession finally accepted that spontaneous generation was wrong. In 1840, Ignatz Semmelweis proved that washing hands saved lives in hospitals but years later during the US Civil War and even for many years after, many American doctors refused to wash their hands calling it a ridiculous waste of time. Today, the refusal of the medical profession to accept certain things causes the deaths of millions each year. Sepsis and septicemia kills millions, far more than AIDS, yet where is the publicity? What improvements have been made? Doctors say that they are concerned about finding the actual cause of AIDS yet when they are presented with reasonable evidence that parasites may be involved, they turn up their noses. This problem reaches to the basic snobbishness of medical doctors in general. Medical doctors are considered elite. Basically, Dr. Clark is only a naturopath, how can she know something that they do not? The FDA has the arrogance to claim that only a drug can cure a disease. Only a doctor can provide a cure to a diseased person. Herbals are nothing more than junk to the FDA which has tried on several occasions to outlaw them. The FDA is currently trying to have vitamins and herbals only available by prescription.

Cryoablation

Extremely cold gas is passed through a needle int a tumor which destroys the tumor by freezing it.

Electrical tumor ablation

Uses electric current that is injected into a tumor using a needle probe to destroy cancer cells within the tumor.

Max Gerson

Many people over the years have looked for a cancer treatment that would have good success without all of the toxic damage that comes from traditional therapy. Especially for people that have time and are not in the very critical late stages, this is a therapy to consider.

It is especially important to consider because it helps to eliminate the cause of cancer rather than taking some toxic drug, hoping that it kills the cancer first before it kills you.

As is normal for the cancer industry, there has been numerous attempts to defame and deride this therapy.

Dr. Max Gerson developed one of the most effective natural cancer treatments over 90 years ago. Known as the "Gerson Therapy," using this therapy, Dr. Gerson helped hundreds of cancer patients boost their body's ability to heal itself by using several techniques, including Organic plant-based foods, Raw juices, Coffee enemas, Beef liver, and Natural supplements.

The Gerson therapy is a whole-body approach to healing that naturally boosts your body's ability to heal without damaging side effects. This immune boosting helps the body to heal cancer, arthritis, heart disease, allergies, as well as other degenerative conditions.

The Gerson Therapy works by targeting the metabolic requirements in your body allowing the patient to benefit from the nutritional consumption of 15–20 pounds of organically grown fruits and vegetables each day. The diet allows eating only organic fruits, vegetables and sprouted ancient grains, and is exceptionally rich in vitamins, minerals and important enzymes. It's also very low in fats, proteins and sodium. The meal plan advises cancer patients to drink 13 glasses of freshly prepared juice, eat three plant-based meals, and only snack on fresh fruits each day. Traditionally, the Gerson Therapy recommends consuming raw beef liver since it is the most nutrient-dense food on the planet and extremely high in vitamin B12.

Freshly pressed juice from raw foods provides the easiest and most effective way of providing high quality nutrition. The protocol calls for patients to drink fresh vegetables each day, including raw carrots or apples and green-leaf juice. To preserve the nutritional content, the juice should be prepared hourly using a two-step juicer or a masticating juicer used with a separate hydraulic press. This helps prevent denaturation — when vitamins, minerals and enzymes are destroyed, often by the heat generated during the juicing process.

Coffee enemas are a primary method of detoxing the body by increasing the parasympathetic nervous system. For cancer patients, up to five enemas a day may be taken.

Once the patient is put on the full therapy, the combined effect of the food, the juices, etc. boosts the immune system allowing it to attack and kill tumor tissue, besides working to flush out accumulated toxins from the body tissues. There is a risk of overburdening and poisoning the liver, which is likely to be already damaged and debilitated.

The Gerson Therapy recommends the additional organic supplements, Lugol's Iodine solution as an additional immune booster and antibiotic, Pancreatic enzymes that help remove the protective protein coating from cancer cells, Potassium compound which is needed for the kidneys to excrete many toxins and is alkalizing as well. Thyroid hormone also helps to boost the immune system, and Vitamin B12. Many patients have had excellent success with the Gerson therapy.

Nicholas J. Gonzalez

The Gonzalez Protocol is a combination diet and supplementation cancer treatment that is specifically supposed to work with pancreatic cancer. In addition to diet and supplementation, the protocol uses other treatments such as enemas, skin brushing, and **baking soda** baths to treat cancer. The protocol has also been used for the treatment of cancers other than pancreatic cancer in addition to other conditions such as chronic fatigue syndrome and multiple sclerosis.

Henderson

This protocol is an adaptation of the Budwig Protocol and is designed to generate an alkaline environment in which microbes cannot thrive. It is based on the point that microbial involvement in cancer development is supported by a growing body of scientific evidence. This cancer diet is intended to establish an unfavorable environment for the progression of cancer and other diseases as well.

While not usually recommended for late stage, aggressive, or advanced cancers, this protocol does have some powerful attributes. This protocol uses the flax seed oil and cottage cheese from the

Budwig protocol to help buy time and to allow less aggressive approaches to be used.

The protocol can produce noticeable effects quickly if the patient has not had chemotherapy but the damage to the immune system caused by chemotherapy can delay benefits. As the protocol is based in building immunity, it has several immune-building products in it, that the patient can choose from. Beta Glucan is suggested as a helpful supplement to support immune function.

Hoffer, Abram

In his notes: Dr. Hoffer suggested that cancer sufferers should obey three rules: (1) To eliminate all junk food, i.e. food containing any added simple sugars like table sugar or glucose as in corn syrup. This simple rule, can eliminate nearly 90% of the additives commonly added to processed foods. (2) To reduce fat levels, especially dairy products. Almost every study internationally has shown that countries with lower fat intake have fewer cases of cancer, particularly breast cancer. Milk is very rich in estrogens from the cow and in phytoestrogens from the grass they eat. (3) To eliminate all foods they know a person knows that they are allergic to. These rules allow the diet to be varied, palatable and interesting.

Hoffer Vitamin Supplements

Hoffer said that it is advisable always to work with a knowledgeable physician. But if they cannot find any physician or orthomolecular nutritionist they should go ahead on their own using the information now readily available on nutrition and vitamin supplements. It is best to advise their doctors what they are doing and which supplements they are using. By listing the vitamins and dose ranges I am not suggesting that every person need to take them all. This is a personal matter based on discussions with the individual's doctor. The vitamin and mineral supplements are compatible with medication and with the diet.

<u>Vitamin C:</u> The dose range is anywhere from 3 to 40 grams daily in three divided doses. If the dose is too high it will not be absorbed by the intestines, will stay in the bowel and act like a laxative causing loose stools and gas, often referred to as bowel tolerance. It is a good laxative. The best dose does not act like a laxative. Forms of vitamin C include the pure ascorbic acid (hydrogen ascorbate), and the mineral salts such as sodium ascorbate (slightly salty in taste), calcium ascorbate (slightly bitter), and other salts often found in combinations of the mineral ascorbates. In large doses it is best used as the powder dissolved in water or one of the juices. He recommends not to use commercial grade vitamin C crystals or powders. Use CP grades as is found in drug stores orkelley health food stores. Contrary to false rumors issued by some hostile critics of mega dose vitamin use, it does not cause kidney stones, does not cause pernicious anemia, and does not cause sterility. A recent suggestion in a letter to Nature, published in England, concluded that more than 500 milligrams of vitamin C daily could cause DNA damage. This was based on one of a possible 20 markers that could have been used which showed no damage and a

21st marker which is seriously questioned. Some of the key scientists in this field criticized these conclusions. My only comment is that if they were correct, why do many patients who take large doses of vitamin C live so much longer?

<u>Vitamin B3:</u> There are two forms. Niacin (as nicotinic acid) lowers cholesterol, elevates high density lipoprotein (HDL) cholesterol and reduces the ravages of heart disease, but causes flushing when it is first taken. The flushing reaction dissipates in time and in most cases is gone or very minor within a matter of weeks. Niacinamide, the other form, has no effect on blood fats (lipids) but is not a vasodilator. There have been seven international conferences on the theme niacin and cancer. This vitamin is an essential component of the enzyme systems that repair broken DNA molecules. The dose ranges from 100 milligrams three times daily to 1000 milligrams three times daily. Several studies in Detroit have found that the response rate of cancer around the head and neck was 10% on radiation alone but increased to 80% when patients were given large doses of niacinamide. Very rarely niacin will cause obstructive jaundice which clears when the niacin is stopped. For details see my book Orthomolecular Medicine for Physicians.

<u>Vitamin E (d alpha tocopherol succinate):</u> This water soluble form has the greatest efficacy in controlling cancer cell growth in the test tube and is the one I recommend should be used. (It is now realized that mixed tocopherols and tocotrienols are better.) The dose ranges from

400 to 1200 International Units daily. Vitamin E is the major fat soluble anti-oxidant in the body and plays a role by decreasing the concentration of free radicals which are thought to be involved in the creation of the cancer. It also decreases the risk of heart disease, thus confirming what was found over fifty years in Ontario by Drs. Wilfrid and Evan Shute.

<u>The Carotenoids:</u> Most people have heard of beta carotene but this is only one of a large number of carotenoids which are present in colored vegetables and fruits such as carrots, beets, tomatoes and greens. The evidence is very powerful that these mixed carotenoids as found in these foods will decrease the incidence of cancer, but there is a question about the efficacy of the pure beta carotene. There is still a vigorous debate about this. Hoffer prefers carrot juice to the beta carotene. Generally it is better to have a large variety of these natural anti cancer factors. Beta carotene is very safe. The only question is whether it is the best form. Only a small portion is converted into vitamin A.

<u>Folic acid:</u> Several studies have found this important vitamin has anti cancer properties, for cancer of the cervix and of the lung in lung smokers. This does not mean it is safe to smoke. It does mean that smokers should take it and immediately start their campaign to stop smoking. Women should take ample amounts to prevent neural tube disorders such as spina bifida. The US government plans to add it to

flour. Canada is still thinking about it. The dose range is from 1 to 30 milligrams daily. It can be taken on prescription.

Coenzyme Q10: Dr. Karl Folkers discovered this substance, also called ubiquinone; toward the end of his long and distinguished career he regretted that he had not called it a vitamin. It is an odd vitamin since young people are able to make enough from the lower numbered ubiquinones such as Q6 or Q8 whereas older people, and anyone ill, are not able to make enough. It thus becomes a vitamin later in life and when one becomes ill. A few clinical studies have shown that in large doses it has anticancer properties especially for breast cancer. These range from 300 milligrams to 600 milligrams daily.

Hoffer Mineral Supplements

Selenium: The presence or absence of this trace element has the clearest relationship to the presence of cancer. People living on soils that are rich in selenium have a lower incidence. I recommend between 200 to 1000 micrograms daily. One of my patients took 2000 mcg with no side effects.

Calcium and Magnesium: These are generally very useful to take to maintain calcium levels in bones and blood. They have been found helpful in cases of bowel cancer. Women should receive 1500 milligrams of calcium daily from their food and supplements, and half as much magnesium. There are several forms of these minerals available. Usually a person will absorb into their body anywhere between 25 and 50% of the calcium.

Zinc and Copper: There is a reciprocal connection between these two. If blood zinc levels are too high the copper levels will be too low. Because zinc can shrink enlarged prostate glands and may be helpful in the treatment of this cancer. I have been using it routinely. Also, people in Victoria tend to be low in zinc levels because our water is soft, and dissolves copper more easily from copper plumbing.

The above was slightly modified from A. Hoffer's original writing.

Hoxey

This protocol uses a tonic that contains barberry, buckthorn bark, burdock root, cascara, licorice, pokeweed, potassium iodide, prickly The above was slightly modified from A. Hoffer's original writing.ash bark, red clover and stillingia root along with a diet that eliminates pork, sugar, and bleached flour. The Hoxsey method also requires such things as iron, salt, calcium, vitamin c, yeast supplements and grape juice to also be avoided. The combination of both the tonic and diet were promoted to eliminate toxins from the body and in-turn correct cell metabolism, blood chemistry, and immune function.
The FDA has outlawed the use of the Hoxsey protocol in the US.

Linda Lee Isaacs

Dr. Issacs, who previously worked with Dr. Nicholas Gonzalez, offers individualized nutritional protocols for patients with cancer and other illnesses, as well as protocols for health maintenance.

immunotherapy uses non-toxic vaccine and cell therapy protocols, which have no adverse side-effects. The vaccine and immune cells are prepared from the patients own body and are specific to the patient.

Kelley

Metabolic **Protocol uses** enzymes to strip the protein coating off of **cancer** cells so the immune system can identify and kill the **cancer** cells. While operating, Dr. **Kelley** and his practitioners treated more 33,000 patients, claiming a 93 percent success rate for those who came to him before chemotherapy, radiation, or surgery, not after any such traditional therapies had been used.

Because the pancreas produces more than 30 enzymes, in addition to insulin, Dr. Kelley considered it to be a key fighter of cancer. Among these enzymes, the proteolytic enzymes were considered to be key in defense of cancer.

Harold Manner

promoted the use of Laetril or vitamin B17 to treat cancer.

Moerman

believed that cancer was the result of a malfunctioning immune system due to nutritional problems.

There are eight key nutrients in this diet:

1) Vitamin A (requires Vitamin D as a catalyst),

2) Vitamin B complex,

3) Vitamin C,

4) Vitamin E,

5) Citric Acid,

6) Iodine,

The above was slightly modified from A. Hoffer's original writing. The above was slightly modified from A. Hoffer's original writing. 7) Iron,

8) Sulphur

Osiecki

protocol is intended to block the 3 steps of metastasis through nutritional factors. In the three steps, the cancer cell must first detach itself from the primary site, then secondly, it must penetrate the normal cell matrix and thirdly, it needs to perforate the surrounding blood vessels for entry and dissemination.

Radio frequency ablation

This process uses the heat and electrical energy injected through a probe into a tumor to locally destroy cancer cells in the tumor.

Mathias Rath

uses a nutrient combination of vitamin C, the amino-acids L-lysine and L-proline, and Epigallocatechin Gallate (EGCG) from green tea.

Carl Reich

In the early 1950's, while pursuing post-graduate studies, began to suspect that a number of imbalances and diseases could be traced to deficiencies of specific vitamins and minerals, in particular, calcium.

Starting about 1954, he began treating his patients with nutritionalThe above was slightly modified from A. Hoffer's original writing. supplements. Patients with a variety of symptoms such as constipation, leg cramps, chronic asthma, and sinusitis experienced rapid relief when treated with elevated calcium and vitamin D, as well as a wide spectrum of basic nutrients.

He then began to treat more patients with his nutritional therapy. A wide range of symptoms such as headaches, muscle pain, constipation, indigestion, and migraines were successfully treated with calcium and other nutrients. He also came to believe that a number of diseases as diverse as chronic arthritis, asthma, Rheumatoid_Arthritis , ileitis and colitis, hypertension, heart spasms, diabetes, Alzheimer's disease, Parkinson's disease, Lou Gehrig's disease, and even cancer, were all in some way related to calcium deficiency. Since the nervous system is highly dependent on calcium, he believed that when the body is under stress, the autonomic nervous system sends out various messages to internal organs and that improper nutrition interferes with this. Through his studies on patients over many years, he saw proof that calcium, magnesium and vitamin D were very often the key factors in disease.

Rife Therapy involves the use of specific frequencies that are user to modulate a RF carrier of electromagnetic energy to treat cancer and other issues as well. It's a non-invasive treatment that was developed in the 1930's by a man named Royal Raymond Rife, an optical engineer and technician. Using a special tool the he designed and built, called the Rife Universal Microscope, Rife was able to observe the microorganism that causes cancer while the microorganism was still alive. As a result, he was then able to build and tune a machine, the Rife Beam Ray to the microorganism's Mortal Oscillatory Rate (MOR). Patients who were treated with the Rife Beam Ray tuned to a MOR specific to the invading pathogen for just a few minutes were often miraculously cured. In fact, several sources from the period reported that the Rife Beam Ray machine had a success rate of higher than 90% at treating cancer.

So, why do we not have this microscope and Beam Ray machines today? Mostly because they were destroyed to keep them from being used in order to keep the pharmaceutical industry profitable.

A couple of the microscopes still exist but are not complete. Since the documentation was destroyed, No one has been able to recreate these marvels. We do know that they did exist and were functional from past reports.

There are some Beam Ray machines available today but they do not meet all of the technical requirements because the original documentation was also destroyed. We do know however that the use of electromagnetic frequencies does work because the FDA has approved certain restricted uses of these types of machines for the treatment of certain cancers, but only after full chemotherapy and radiation procedures have been followed.

The use of these machines is not generally a good application for use in the doctor's office as they require frequent and extensive usage for full effect.

A quick note from Dr. Schulze's own website:

"Since I had so many patients with cancer, I decided to do this same research and discovered the exact same scenario and statistics.

I discovered that the group that died the quickest, from various types of cancer, was the group who did the most aggressive medical treatments. In fact, the speed at which patients died from cancer was usually totally equal to the aggressiveness of their medical therapy. **I discovered that the group that lived longer** was the group who did nothing at all for their cancer. They lived longer and also had a much better quality of life. They just totally ignored the cancer, rotted away and eventually died, but they lived happier, healthier, had less pain (if any), had a better quality of life and lived quite a bit longer. Some even recovered."

SCMT

or Systemic Cancer Multistep Therapy, developed by Manfred von Ardenne. was based on the Warburg Effect. The process basically overloads the cancer cells with lactic acid and then forces apoptosis through generating a hig fever. Glucose is injected into the blood over the course of about 30 hours which causes the pH of cancer cells to drop to around 5.5 from the excess lactic acid produced. The patient then sits in an area heated to about 104 degrees Fahrenheit. The time that a patient spends in the hot environment depends on their age. The patient is allowed to breathe cool air while their body is heated. This treatment is intended to kill the low-pH cancer cells while stabilizing and detoxifying normal, healthy cells at the same time.

Diathermy (heating the body with high-frequency electrical currents) is used locally to further cause the temperature of tumors to rise to 106 degrees Fahrenheit or higher. Diathermy allows only a localized area of the body in and around the tumor to be heated to 106 degrees. The high temperature combined with an acidic environment inside the cell shortens the life of a cancer cell.

recommends using baking soda as a cancer treatment and it is oriented mostly towards cancers of the digestive tract. He lost his license and there is not much support for his therapy. That, however, does not mean that it doesn't work.

uses heat to destroy cancers tissue and cells.

was awarded a Nobel Prize for was for making the discovery that low oxygen was characteristic of cancer cells. Warburg did hypothesize that oxygen might be used to cure cancer, but when he tried to cure cancer with oxygen, he failed. Later in his years he became convinced that illness such as cancer resulted from pollution.

recommended consuming wheatgrass juice and other live foods to fight cancer while at the same time, avoiding all meat, dairy products and cooked foods.

Are generally portable devices designed to partially replace technologies such as Rife Machines and these devices range from primitive single frequency units that are very cheap to more advanced multi-frequency machines. Some of these are based on the work done by Royal Rife and John Crane in the 1950's and provide multiple frequencies with the convenience of pad contact with high accuracy.

In my opinion, the real value of a zapper is in fighting infections because 9 percent of cancer sufferers die of infection and a good zapper can make a difference in survival and longevity.

The following books are recommended.

"Death by Diet" by Robert R. Barefoot

"The Cure for All Cancers" by Dr. Hulda Clark, Ph.D., N.D.

"Disease Prevention and Treatment" Life Extension Foundation

"Lung Cancer: Myths, Facts, Choices – and Hope" by Claudia Henschke, et al

"Natural Cures They Don't Want You to Know About" by Kevin Trudeau

"Remarkable Recovery" by Caryle Hirshberg, Marc Ian Barasch

"Liver and Cancer" by Casper Blond

For those interested in Biology or Electro-Biology:

"The Body Electric" by Dr. Robert O. Becker, M.D.

"Cross Currents" by Dr. Robert O. Becker, M.D.

For further information visit these web sites.

www.cancertutor.com

www.lef.org

www.paradevices.com/cancer.html

www.curezone.com/diseases/cancer

www.mendosa.com

www.unitogether.com

www.hulda-clark-quack.com

Peoples with low cancer rates

In the remote recesses of the Himalayan Mountains, between West Pakistan, India and China there is a tiny Kingdom called Hunza. These people are known world over for their amazing longevity and health. They live well beyond 100 years and have commonly been known to still father children at the age of 110. One of the first medical teams to study the Hunza was headed by world-renown British surgeon Dr Robert McCarrison. In the AMA Journal Jan 7, 1922 he reported:

"The Hunza has no known incidence of cancer. They have an abundant crop of apricots. These they dry in the sun and use largely in their food".

It is interesting to note that the traditional Hunza Diet contains over 200 times more nitriloside (B17 Rich food) than the average American or Australian Diet. There is no such thing as money in Hunza. A mans wealth is measured by the number of apricot trees he owns. And the most prized of all foods was considered to be the apricot seed. It is very common for the Hunza to eat between 30 - 50 (ie. about 30mg of B17) apricot seeds as an after lunch snack. The thousands of seeds they do not eat they store or grind them very finely and then squeezed under pressure to produce a very rich oil used in cooking and to apply to the skin. The apricot is staple food in Hunza. They use the apricot, its seed and the oil for practically everything. In addition to the ever present apricot, the hunzahuts eat mainly grain and fresh vegetables. These include buckwheat, millet, alfalfa, peas, broad beans, turnips, lettuce, sprouting pulse and berries of various sorts. All of these with the exception of lettuce and turnips contain vitamin B17.

It is important to know when the Hunza leave their secluded land and adopt the menus of other countries, they soon succumb to the same diseases and infirmities including cancer as the rest of man kind.

ESKIMOS

The Eskimos are another people that have been observed by medical teams for many decades and found to be totally free of cancer. The traditional Eskimo diet is amazingly rich in B17 nitrilosides that come from the residue of of the meat of caribou and other grazing animals, and also from the salmon berry. Another Eskimo delicacy is green salad made out of the stomach contents of caribou and reindeer which are full of fresh tundra grass. Tundra grasses such as Arrow are have shown to be contain the highest content of B17 than other grasses.

Alaska's most famous doctor Dr Preston A Price claims that, "In his 36 years of contact with these people he had never seen a single case of malignant disease among the truly primitive Eskimos, although it frequently occurred when they were modernized.

An interesting point to note is that when an Eskimo leaves his traditional way of life and begins to rely on a western/modern diet he becomes even more cancer prone than the average American.

HOPI & NAVAJO INDIANS

The Indians of North America are another people who are remarkably free from cancer. The AMA went as far as conducting a special study in an effort to discover why there was little to no cancer amongst the Hopi and Navajo Indians. The February 5, 1949 issue of the journal of the American Medical Association declared that they found 36 cases cases of malignant cancer from a population of 30,000. In the same population of white persons there would have been about 1800. Dr Krebs research later found that the typical diet for the Navajo and Hopi Indian consisted of nitriloside-rich foods such as Cassava. He calculated that some of the tribes would ingest the equivalent of 8000mg of Vitamin B17 per day from their diet !!!

ABKHAZIANS

The Abkhazians are found deep in the Caucasus Mountains on the Northwest side of the Black Sea. They are a people with almost the exact same health record and longevity as the Hunzakuts. Their food and lifestyle having to live in a harsh rugged terrain are almost identical. They follow a diet which is low in carbohydrates, high in vegetable proteins and rich in minerals and vitamins, especially vitamin B17.

Signs of cancer

1. Wheezing or shortness of breath

Often found as an early sign in lung cancer patients is that they remember noticing when they look back is the inability to catch their breath.

2. Chronic cough or chest pain

Some cancers, including leukemia and lung tumors, can cause symptoms that mimic a bad cough or bronchitis. Especially true if the problems persist, or go away and come back again in a repeating cycle. Occasionally, lung cancer patients may report chest pain that extends up into the shoulder or down the arm.

3. Frequent fevers or infections

This can be a sign of weakened immunity and possibly a sign of leukemia which causes the marrow to produce abnormal white blood cells, crowding out healthy white cells, reducing the body's infection-fighting capabilities.

4. Difficulty swallowing

This is frequently associated with esophageal or throat cancer, having trouble swallowing is sometimes an early sign of lung cancer.

5. Swollen lymph nodes or lumps on the neck, groin, or under the arms

Enlarged lymph nodes usually indicate changes in the lymphatic system, which can be a sign of cancer or other immunity issues. A lump or an enlarged lymph node under the arm can be a sign of breast cancer. Also, a painless lump on the neck, groin, or under the arm can be an early sign of leukemia.

6. Excessive bruising or bleeding that doesn't stop

This sometimes suggests something abnormal happening with the platelets and red blood cells, which can be a sign of leukemia.

7. Weakness and fatigue

Fatigue and weakness is a symptom of so many different kinds of cancer and also other conditions that you'll need to look at it in combination with other symptoms. But any time you feel exhausted without explanation and it doesn't respond to getting more sleep, talk to your doctor.

8. Bloating or abdominal weight gain

Sudden or continued bloating that is beyond what is normally experienced may be a real cause for concern.

9. Feeling full and unable to eat

A loss of appetite can be a concern and if you can't eat even when you haven't eaten for some time should raise an alarm.

10. Pelvic or abdominal pain

Because it's a common symptom of fibroids, ovarian cysts, and other reproductive tract disorders, doctors don't always think of cancer when you describe pelvic pain. Make sure your doctor looks at all possible causes. If the spleen is enlarged, this may be a sign of Leukemia.

11. Rectal bleeding or blood in stool

Blood in the toilet alone is reason to call your doctor and schedule a colonoscopy. However, think back over the last few meals, did you eat beets or some other food that is strongly red in color? Did you eat food with red dye such as "red hots"? If it is blood or even streaks of black in your stool, have it checked.

12. Unexplained weight loss

If you are losing weight unexpectedly and you haven't made changes to your diet or exercise regime, you need to ask why. Weight loss is an early sign digestive tract cancers and possibly a sign of cancer that's spread to the liver.

13. Upset stomach or stomachache

Aching in the abdominal area is not good, especially if persistent or frequently repeating. A quick visit to the doctor may catch something in time to save your life.

14. Red, sore, or swollen breast or nipple changes

Cellulite-like dimpled skin on an area of the breast or red inflamed areas of the breast may be taken as a warning, in addition to lumps. Also a nipple that began to appear flattened, inverted, or turned sideways or becomes crusty, itchy, or scaly. Also if a breast feels warmer than normal. Ask your doctor to prescribe a thermographic breast exam rather than a mammogram. The new modern thermography is far improved and does not subject you to cancer causing radiation.

15. Unusually heavy or painful periods or bleeding between periods

Endometrial or uterine cancer is often initially overlooked by many doctors. Request a transvaginal ultrasound if you suspect something more than routine heavy periods.

16. Swelling of facial features

Puffiness, swelling, or redness in the face can be a sign of some cancers such as lung cancer.

17. A sore or skin lump that doesn't heal, becomes crusty, or bleeds easily

In addition to changes in moles or even freckles, other signs, such as small waxy lumps or dry scaly patches, are easier to miss. Check the skin all over the body for odd-looking growths or spots and be familiar with the different types of skin cancer — melanoma, basal cell carcinoma, and squamous cell carcinoma.

18. Changes in nails

The fingernails can be a indicator of several types of cancer. If the nail beds are pale or white, this is usually a sign of liver problems. Brown or black streaks or dots under the nail can indicate skin cancer. Clubbing or enlargement of the ends of the fingers, with nails that curve down over the tips can be a sign of lung cancer.

19. Pain in the back or lower right side

Liver cancer, ovarian cancer, and even breast cancer can cause back pain. Pain in the lower back may be a sign of kidney issues.

Alphabetical Index

THERAPIES AND PROTOCOLS...123

THE FOLLOWING BOOKS ARE RECOMMENDED...152